Governing Home Care

GLOBALIZATION AND WELFARE

Series Editors: Denis Bouget, *MSH Ange Guépin, France* and Jane Lewis, *Professor of Social Policy, London School of Economics, UK*

This important series is designed to make a significant contribution to the principles and practice of comparative social policy. It includes both theoretical and empirical work. International in scope, it addresses issues of current and future concern in both East and West, and in developed and developing countries.

The main purpose of this series is to create a forum for the publication of high quality work to help understand the impact of globalization on the provision of social welfare. It offers state-of-the-art thinking and research on important areas such as privatization, employment, work, finance, gender and poverty. It includes some of the best theoretical and empirical work from both well established researchers and the new generation of scholars.

Titles in the series include:

The Third Sector in Europe
Edited by Adalbert Evers and Jean-Louis Laville

The OECD and European Welfare States
Edited by Klaus Armingeon and Michelle Beyeler

Poverty and Subsidiarity in Europe
Minimum Protection from an Economic Perspective
Didier Fouarge

Gender Divisions and Working Time in the New Economy
Changing Patterns of Work, Care and Public Policy in Europe and North America
Edited by Diane Perrons, Colette Fagan, Linda McDowell, Kath Ray and Kevin Ward

Social Policy, Employment and Family Change in Comparative Perspective
Edited by Jonathan Bradshaw and Aksel Hatland

Governing Home Care
A Cross-National Comparison
Viola Burau, Hildegard Theobald and Robert H. Blank

Governing Home Care

A Cross-National Comparison

Viola Burau

Associate Professor in Public Policy, University of Aarhus, Denmark

Hildegard Theobald

Professor of Organisational Gerontology and Social Services, University of Vechta, Germany

Robert H. Blank

Research Scholar, New College of Florida, Sarasota, Florida, USA and Visiting Professor, University of Canterbury, Christchurch, New Zealand

GLOBALIZATION AND WELFARE

Edward Elgar

Cheltenham, UK • Northampton, MA, USA

Published by
Edward Elgar Publishing Limited
Glensanda House
Montpellier Parade
Cheltenham
Glos GL50 1UA
UK

Edward Elgar Publishing, Inc.
William Pratt House
9 Dewey Court
Northampton
Massachusetts 01060
USA

A catalogue record for this book
is available from the British Library

Library of Congress Cataloging in Publication Data

Burau, Viola Desideria.
Governing home care : a cross-national comparison / by Viola Burau, Hildegard Theobald, Robert H. Blank.
p. cm. — (Globalization and welfare series)
Includes bibliographical references and index.
1. Older people—Services for—Case studies. 2. Older people—Home care—Case studies. 3. Caregivers—Case studies. 4. Social policy—Case studies. I. Theobald, Hildegard. II. Blank, Robert H. III. Title.
HV1451.B86 2007
362.6'3—dc22

2007000150

ISBN 978 1 84542 752 8

Printed and bound in Great Britain by MPG Books Ltd, Bodmin, Cornwall

Contents

Figures

Tables

Acknowledgements

This book has been a complex project in many ways, involving a comparison across nine countries and four substantive areas of governing home care written by three researchers who work and live in four countries spread across three continents. In the process of managing this complexity, we have greatly benefited from the support of our respective universities and our colleagues in the field. The Programme for International Guest Researchers at the University of Aarhus funded two research stays of two and six months, respectively, which gave us valuable opportunities for face-to-face discussions. The Department of Political Science at the university provided not only excellent office facilities but also an inspiring research environment. The Danish National Institute of Social Research in Copenhagen funded a research stay for two of us during the crucial final phase of the project, and we would like to thank especially Tine Rostgaard for making this possible. A research stay funded by the Institute for Future Studies in Stockholm provided one of us with the opportunity to conduct research and to discuss our concepts and findings in Sweden. We would like to thank Joakim Palme for this invitation.

The wide range of countries included in the analysis has also made it necessary to work with country experts in relation to areas less well covered in the international literature. In particular, we would like to thank the following individuals: Giovanni Lamura (Italian National Research Centre on Ageing, Ancona) for valuable additions to our analysis of Italy and for writing a case study on the development of the Italian approach on home care and its political and socio-economic background; Hannerieke van der Boom (University of Maastricht) for letting us use a chapter on the Netherlands from her forthcoming comparative study of home nursing; Karel de Bakker and Trudie Knijn (University of Utrecht) for writing the case study on the policy development related to the introduction of personal budgets in the Netherlands; Sirli Kivisaar and Annely Soots (Estonian Association of Gerontology and Geriatrics, Tartu) for their comprehensive report on the development of social and health care in Estonia which formed the basis for our analysis of the Estonian situation; Marta Szebehely and Gun-Britt Trydegard (University of Stockholm) for providing us with valuable information and for discussions on the development of social care services and support systems for the elderly in Sweden; Stina-Clara Hjulström, president of the Dementia Association in Sweden, for her inspiring interview on processes of policy development in Sweden; and David Feltenius (University of Umeå) for sending us his dissertation on the political influence of the pensioners' organisations in Sweden.

We have presented individual parts of the book at a range of conferences and research seminars and we were lucky to receive many comments that were both challenging and constructive. Here we would like to mention in particular the research seminars at the Feminist Research Centre at Aalborg University and at the Danish National Institute for Social Research in Copenhagen, and the sessions on users and care workers at the ISA World Congress of Sociology in Durban, South Africa. At the World Congress in Durban, Meri Koivusalo (National Research and Development Centre for Welfare and Health, STAKES, Finland) commented constructively and inspiringly on a part of our book. At the University of Aarhus, Mette Nørgaard Andersen provided invaluable research assistance at different points of the project and Lone Winther carefully edited our bibliography.

Viola Burau
Hildegard Theobald
Robert H. Blank

1. Introduction to the governance of home care

This chapter introduces home care as a complicated set of activities that transcend a number of boundaries, especially between public and private, formal and informal, and the micro and the macro levels. We discuss the importance of defining care by its location and provide an overview of the different locations that are used to define 'home', as well as the dynamics between different home locations. This chapter also introduces the concept of 'governance' as applied to home care, and introduces the close relationship between the public/private and the formal and informal sectors.[1] It demonstrates that the governance of home care has become highly politicised because of demographic developments relating to ageing populations, societal developments relating to individualisation and changing gender cultures, including changes in the traditional role of families as care givers, and economic developments relating to heightened resource constraints across all policy areas.

This chapter also explains our choice of countries for analysis and offers an overview of the relevant cultural and institutional contexts of home care in each country, which are fleshed out in Chapter 3.[2] Finally we introduce the issue of convergence. At the theoretical level there is currently considerable debate between those who argue that there is a convergence of policy across countries and others who contend that despite convergence, in some arenas there remains considerable divergence due to cultural and structural variation. These latter observers point to the embeddedness of policies in country-specific contexts. Home care governance across these countries serves as an excellent test of the convergence hypothesis.

DEFINING HOME CARE

The user groups of home care are diverse and reflect the support required at different stages of the life span, ranging from severely ill infants to people at the end of their life. Other beneficiaries of home care include people with mental illness and handicap, physical disability, drug-related disorders and progressive illness (Means et al., 2003). Each of these groups raises a different set of issues and problems. Thus to provide a workable focus, this book deals exclusively with home care for older people. Already older people constitute by far the largest user group of home care, a figure that will increase significantly in the light of the ageing of societies, discussed in more detail below.

We use Tester's definition of home care as 'any type of care and support offered to older people in their homes, whether ordinary or specialised settings, by formal and informal carers' (1996: 76). Home care thus encompasses a wide range of tasks and activities, and cuts across the boundaries between health and social care and between formal and informal care. It includes basic mobility and self-care, medical and nursing care to help with physical and mental health problems, help in daily living tasks, counselling and emotional support to promote well-being; as well as other social, educational and leisure activities (Tester, 1996). Home care usually involves nurses rather than doctors, as well as home helps and most importantly women as informal carers. Indeed, unpaid carers deliver most home care, and it is estimated that formal care comprises only one-fifth of the total help older people receive (Jacobzone, 1999). The diversity of care subsumed under home care reflects the disparate yet interlocking needs of people who require long-term care. Diversity makes such care interesting but also difficult to define, analyse and compare. Moreover, care services are often locally specific and even tailored to particular individuals, and it is difficult to identify the typical case let alone to generalise.

Home care, then, is a highly complex activity that includes not only a wide range of different tasks but also transcends the distinction between formal services and informal relationships. The former links home care governance to the dynamics of policy making and different approaches to governing, whereas the latter links home care governance to the wider family and gender structures in society. Informal care in turn can be delivered by trained professionals, untrained and often poorly paid helpers, family or friends. Home care also crosses the boundaries between the domestic and public life and the macro and micro levels. The boundary between public and private which is evident in more traditional policy areas is blurred in home care. Although some of these services might be provided formally through an array of public and private organisational structures, much home care is informal and thus outside the purview of formal controls, often provided by friends or relatives without any regularised rules of guidance. Home care also obscures the distinction between the macro and micro levels and introduces a tension between hierarchical and individualistic approaches. Because it can be so multifaceted and decentralised, home care requires analysis at both levels simultaneously.

Chapter 3 examines in more detail the interface between formal and informal care and the underpinning cultural expectations about the role of women in care giving. This linkage is important because, as acknowledged by recent policy initiatives in many countries, most home care continues to be provided by unpaid carers, primarily women. However, under the banner of greater welfare mix, the objectives of reforms are to integrate carers more explicitly into formal care arrangements and to support carers through payments and related benefits.

Likewise, the line between home and institutional care remains an ambiguous one. In the US and to a lesser extent other countries, assisted-care living facilities have been initiated that combine the two concepts. Usually the facility has three levels of care depending on the health and mobility of the older person. Homes and apartments in the independent care section allow those who need particular care services to get them. As they need more extensive care they move into a room or apartment that provides a more intensive care environment. And finally, they can move to a nursing home facility located in the same complex. In the US, these care facilities are a mix of for-profit (usually more high-end facilities) and non-profit (often church or charity based). The point here, though, is that while the literature conceptually distinguishes home from institutional care, in reality this distinction is blurred. With this caveat in mind, however, our analysis will focus on the location of care in the home setting.

FRAMEWORK FOR STUDYING THE GOVERNANCE OF HOME CARE

In order to structure our analysis of governing home care in a helpful manner we have constructed the framework in Figure 1.1. Because home care crosses many traditional boundaries in public policy analysis (formal/informal, public/private, macro/micro) this book addresses the concept of governance instead of the more traditionally studied public policy. This allows us to account for the complexity of home care where public policy is but one element. We contend that to understand home care governance we must examine all the relevant institutions and ideas as well as actors. In terms of institutions we shall analyse social institutions (especially relating to gender arrangements), political institutions (including sector-specific institutional arrangements, but also broader institutional arrangements such as the welfare state and the political system), and the opportunities and constraints institutions make in relation to governance options. Finally, in terms of ideas we analyse culturally embedded traditions, beliefs and attitudes relating to home care and the changing nature of ideas (as reflected in 'critical instances' that introduce new ideas and help to account for changing governing arrangements).

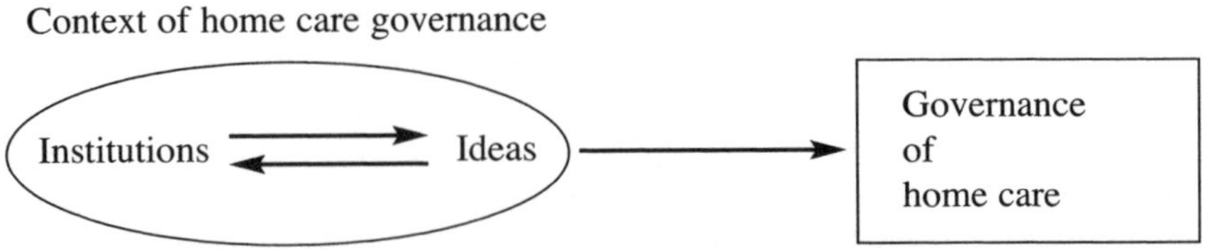

Figure 1.1 Framework for analysing the governance of home care

This analytical framework aims to map out and differentiate among the many ways in which the governance of home care comes about. It is used to map out home care and its organisation and to account for differences and similarities across countries by analysing relevant ideas and institutions and the interplay between them. There are many processes (understood as interactions between institutions and ideas) which shape the governance of home care but which do not go through the formal policy process. This infers that a significant degree of governing goes on beyond government.

Where appropriate, our analysis also looks at explicit processes of policy making. This involves examining the many actors involved, both veto/status quo actors and policy entrepreneurs. The first type is likely to try to keep home care off the political agenda while the second type can be crucial in putting home care on the political agenda. Moreover, these actors can come from within government or from outside. It is also important to note that policy here has two dimensions and entails both specific home care policies and other policies that impact on home care. Because home care transcends many areas, the second dimension is of special relevance in the absence of a dedicated home care policy. In fact we shall see that direct governance through specific policies has been the exception.

It should be emphasised here that despite the directional arrow in our model, it is not meant to describe causal relations but instead characterises a loose and flexible configuration of factors that shape the governance of home care. With many factors operating in each country, the effect of individual factors depends as well on the interplay among them, thus obscuring the formulation of any precise predictions. Despite this caveat, we feel that this framework is valuable in making sense of home care governance across our countries.

As noted earlier, our focus here is on a comprehensive notion of governance of home care rather than public policy in the more restrictive sense. We argue that to understand home care one must analyse different logics of governance (state, associations, market, family) as well as different instruments of governance (delivery, funding and rules) that taken together gives us a four-by-three table that will be used for comparison of the countries (Table 1.1). This more inclusive, and we argue accurate, view of the governance of home care demonstrates that in order to understand differences and similarities of home care across countries we must be aware of the activity not only by the state, but also by associations, the marketplace and the family. Moreover, the instruments of governance will vary not only by locale but also across time, thus explicating the dynamics of home care governance. Chapter 2 will provide more details on the logics and instruments of governance drawn from the literatures of social care and public policy and fill in the blank spaces in Table 1.1.

Table 1.1 Logics and instruments of home care governance (1)

Logics of governance	Instruments of governance		
	Funding	Delivery	Rules
State			
Associations			
Market			
Family			

Governance, then, is an umbrella concept covering a broad range of mechanisms for creating order among different actors in the public sector. Governance moves beyond the purely private to collective action. 'Among the issues which governance invites one to analyse are the relationships among local, regional and national levels, the role of the state and its relationship to civil society, the (re)positioning of different interest groups and the framing, orientation and implementation of policies' (Daly, 2003: 115). Moreover, the locale and exercise of power are central to governance and it is especially attuned to the changing set of arrangements between the state and the other logics. As noted by Jessop (1999), the state is more than a political agent; it is also the bearer of certain types of social packages. This latter is a role that is changing as the welfare state shrinks and globalisation intensifies.

As suggested in the discussion of the analytical framework above, there are two routes to governance of home care, a direct route and an indirect one where the policy process acts as a filter. Although we emphasise a comprehensive analysis of the varied logics, the core intervening variable in home care governance is public policy defined here as an action (or non-action) taken by the government or on behalf of it (Heywood, 1997). It is a goal-driven course of action designed to promote, maintain or prevent a particular state of affairs. While other organisations such as medical associations and care societies often make decisions that affect many individuals as well as the home care system, only the government has the legitimate authority to make decisions that are binding and carried out in the name of the people as a whole.

Home care policy is defined here as those courses of action or non-action proposed or taken by a government that impact on the financing, delivery or rule of home care services. However, while attention is understandably focused on the government, we argue that inclusion of the other logics of governance, including the actions by private and voluntary organisations, the market and the family that impact on home care governance are crucial in crossing the boundaries between public and private dimensions. In some countries, state non-action in the home care arena has been a more common approach than action. Also critical is the fact that although home care conceptually can be distinguished from other areas of public policy, in reality it is highly interrelated with social and economic policy in general. Thus home care policy cannot be understood in isolation from social welfare, health, unemployment, poverty, housing and general economic policies. Therefore where relevant we bring these other policy areas into our analysis.

COMPARATIVE HOME CARE GOVERNANCE

In order to elucidate the similarities and differences in approach among various countries' efforts to resolve similar problems and govern home care, this book places home care governance in a comparative context. Although it is dangerous to apply uncritically policies that work in one county to those in another, comparative policy analysis is useful in expanding policy options and demonstrating the experiences of a wide range of applications. Antonnen et al. (2003a), for instance, conclude that 'current patterns of globalisation in politics, economics and culture and the growing movements of people across borders have raised the significance of comparative social research' (2003: 7). Ovretveit (1998) adds that travel and new information systems are making it both easier and more necessary to understand cultural and national differences. Harrop agrees that 'by examining policies comparatively, we can discover how countries vary in the policies they adopt, gain insight into why these differences exist, and identify some of the conditions under which policies succeed or fail' (1992: 3). Ham (1997: 50) contends that an examination of international experience is illuminating in demonstrating both the difficulties faced by and the wide range of approaches available to policy makers, both public and private.

Comparative studies, then, can give us cross-cultural insights as to governance of home care under a wide variety of institutional and value contexts. For instance, which countries have taken a pro-active approach by making and implementing specific home care policy and which have deferred governance to associations, the market or the family? Given the complexity of governing home care, we argue that only comparative studies can generate the evidence necessary to consider the full array of options.

Comparative analysis can also illustrate the commonalities of problems and variables across countries. Although to some extent home care governance is unique to each nation, one cannot ignore the globalisation of problems and potential solutions. These global forces are seen by some as supporting the *convergence theory*, which argues that as countries industrialise they tend to converge towards the same policy mix (Bennett, 1991). Bolstered by globalisation, the convergence thesis suggests that home care governance across disparate country environments will have a tendency to become more similar over time as they develop economically. Gibson and Means (2000), for example, argue that recent restructuring has led to convergence of the long-term care regimes of Australia and the UK, despite quite dissimilar goals and strategic emphases.

Critics of convergence theories, however, argue that they oversimplify the process of development and underestimate significant divergence across countries (Guillén, 2001, Howlett and Ramesh, 2003: 107). They argue that convergence downplays the importance of country-specific factors other than economic development and that most studies that find evidence of convergence do not find it applicable across the board, thus allowing for divergence in other areas. We also surmise that because home care deals with less standardised, more personalised services often at the local level, any forces of convergence apparent at national levels are likely to be marginalised or at least less consistent than in more formal policy areas. At the least, home care would seem more resistant to convergence than, for instance, health care. Although this book is not designed to test the convergence theory directly, its current prominence in the literature dictates that where appropriate its assumptions be addressed in the following chapters and that its explanatory power across these countries be explored more fully.

COUNTRIES SELECTED FOR ANALYSIS

In order to provide a useful cross-country analysis of home care governance, we selected nine countries for primary coverage. These countries were chosen to give the reader systematic exposure to the full range of institutional and cultural contexts. Although they are all developed countries they differ widely in terms of institutions, ideas and associated actor combinations, and as such they represent a wide spectrum of political, cultural and economic environments for governing home care.[3] The group of case countries includes some such as Germany, Sweden, the Netherlands, the UK and the US that are often included in comparative studies of Western nations, and others such as Estonia, Italy, Japan and New Zealand that are seldom included.[4] Individually, each of the countries has unique contributions to make to the study of home care governance. In combination, these countries serve as a constructive sample upon which to analyse the dynamics of home care governance in the twenty-first century.

Our model suggests that home care governance in any country at a particular point in time is the product of a multitude of factors, including the intrinsic social, cultural and political fabric of a country, which encompass social values and structures, political institutions and traditions, the legal system, and characteristics of the health and social care communities. These institutions and ideas (and actors) can influence home care governance directly or be shaped and filtered through the policy process. For that portion of home care governance impacted on by the policy process it is crucial to understand the characteristics of that process in each country (Anttonen et al., 2003a: 174). For instance policy-making authority can be highly centralised or widely dispersed across multiple levels. Moreover in some countries, unions and/or corporate structures are strong factors in determining social policy and might in effect have a veto power over proposed policy changes made by the government.

Contrasting Political Systems

Although the political systems of no two countries are identical and each nation has a unique combination of formal and informal structures, the characteristics of political systems can be categorised along several overlapping dimensions (Lijphart, 1999). The major distinguishing factor is the extent to which political power is concentrated or dispersed. As a rule, *unitary* systems concentrate political authority in a central government while *federal* systems constitutionally divide powers between the central government and states, provinces or other subnational levels. Although the central government in a unitary system might choose to delegate specific administrative functions and responsibilities to lower units, final authority rests at the national level. In contrast, states in a federal system have constitutionally-based powers that very often include health and social welfare policy. Most European countries have unitary systems while Germany, the Netherlands, and the US are examples of the federal model.

Another institutional configuration that relates directly to the continuum of centralisation is the distribution of power within each level of government. On the one hand many democracies, such as New Zealand and the UK, concentrate power in parliament where the distinction between executive and legislative power is obscured or virtually non-existent. In stark contrast to other countries examined here is the US, with its deliberate constitutional separation of powers among a separately elected president, two houses of Congress and a relatively active judicial system. Despite a great deal of variation in the diffusion of policy-making authority in some parliamentary systems as compared to the US, they all display considerably more concentrated bases of power. Figure 1.2 presents a rough distribution of our case countries in terms of centralisation of institutional power along these dimensions. This distribution corresponds closely to the findings of Lijphart (1999: 189), who classifies Germany and the US as 'federal and decentralised'; the Netherlands as 'semi-federal'; Japan and Sweden as 'unitary and decentralised'; and Italy, New Zealand, Estonia and the UK as 'unitary and centralised'.

Estonia Italy Japan Germany
New Zealand UK Sweden Netherlands US

Concentrated ———————————————— Fragmented

Figure 1.2 Institutional power in political systems

The implications of these formal government types for home care governance are likely to be significant. Where power is highly centralised, the government has the formal capacity to make more rapid and comprehensive policy changes. In contrast, the more fragmented the political authority the greater the probability of deadlock and inaction or at best more incremental change. Moreover, in fragmented political systems where competing political parties are able to control particular institutions, there is more likely to be a divided government where one party controls one or several branches or levels and the other party controls others. Although this might contribute towards a more deliberative policy-making process, it can also degenerate into stagnation and gridlock as has been commonplace in the US. Conversely, it might be expected that a highly centralised system such as the UK or Italy produces a policy arena characterised by more frequent and inclusive changes such as major restructuring, often to the detriment of programme stability.

The most obvious dimension of the political context consists of the formal institutions that have been created for making public policy decisions and which define the distribution of power and the relationships among the political players. As such they give distinct advantages or disadvantages to various groups in society. Equally important to understanding governance are the informal practices and structures that have evolved within a particular formal institutional framework. These traditions and rules of the game define a different political logic in each country. They, too, are critical to the environment within which interest groups, political parties, bureaucrats and individual politicians vie for influence over policy. Together, these formal and informal political institutions shape how politics is conducted and create a strategic context for political conflict within the policy arena. 'Political factors help to determine whether a problem is defined as a public policy that requires action, they shape the way in which the problem is defined, and they intervene in the resolution of that problem' (Immergut, 1992: 10). Although institutional variables are not the only ones that matter, variation in institutional conditions across countries yields different opportunities for the actors involved in policy making in each country (Timmermans, 2001: 311).

The Social, Cultural and Historical Context of Home Care

Each country also brings to home care governance a unique combination of social institutions, and historical and cultural factors that are crucial in explaining its proclivities and characteristics. For instance, political culture is the complex of beliefs, values and attitudes held by the public concerning the proper role of government. To what extent is home care a public as opposed to a private good and, if a public good, on what grounds should it be distributed to individuals? What is the perceived role of the state as opposed to the citizen? In home care especially these cultural differences have broad implications for gender because of the fact that women traditionally have been the primary care givers to the elderly. Likewise, any differences in how societies define the roles of women are likely to impact directly on home care. In order to provide a basis for more in-depth comparison throughout later chapters, we now look briefly at the key defining cultural characteristics that might influence home care, gendered ways in which the individual in society relates to the whole. Table 1.2 shows a rough distribution of these countries as to whether they are classified primarily as communitarian, egalitarian or individualistic cultures.

Countries with communitarian traditions based in either the family or other groupings have designed various mechanisms to ensure the interests of the

Table 1.2 Distribution by type of cultural framework

Communitarian	Egalitarian	Individualistic
Germany	Sweden	US
Netherlands	New Zealand	
Japan	UK	
Estonia		
Italy		

various communities involved in home care. In contrast, egalitarian cultures, although representing divergent political systems, all place emphasis on the entitlement to a range of home care services and on a societal commitment to provide such care on those grounds. On the other hand the US, with its rugged individualism, elevates the individual right to be left alone – for example, not to have to pay for such services through taxes – above the welfare of the community and largely sees home care as an individual or private responsibility. As such, the different cultural frameworks of home care are also highly gendered, with communitarian and individualistic frameworks relying heavily on unpaid female labour of love (by design and default, respectively) while the egalitarian framework largely treats such care as a public responsibility. Although rights and entitlements are often used synonymously, entitlements suggest a concern for equality that can be found only in the notion of positive rights. In contrast, the individualistic version of negative, self-centred rights lacks the social dimension found in egalitarian and communitarian societies. A brief look at the most defining characteristics of each of our countries will put this in perspective.

Germany

Germany has a strong tradition of voluntarism, self-help and family support embedded in Roman Catholic social teachings and the idea of 'subsidiarity'. The 1873 social health insurance, the first of its kind, built on these traditions and incorporated them in a statutory system of social solidarity (Freeman, 2000). The organisation of social health care in Germany is marked by profound continuity and is shaped by a number of principles, among them social solidarity, freedom of choice and nearly full coverage of services (Greiner and Schulenburg, 1997). Since 1995, even long-term care needs are covered by a compulsory social insurance. In contrast to social health insurance, however, the long-term care insurance is oriented towards basic needs only. In the context of the social insurance, access to health/social care is an entitlement that individuals 'earn' by virtue of paying insurance contributions. This, together with a strong legalistic approach typical of Germany, turns access to care into the right of individuals to a defined range of services. Individuals literally have 'ownership' of these services or cash benefits. The individualised right to health care also goes hand in hand with the expectation that the social health insurance provides full coverage.

The Netherlands

Another example of a communitarian country is the Netherlands, which resembles Germany in that private initiative has been a guiding principle in the organisation of society. Dutch society has traditionally been organised in separate segments or 'pillars' that represent different religious and political orientations. According to the Roman Catholic notion of subsidiarity and its Protestant counterpart of sovereignty, the different segments in society are to be empowered to provide for their members (Björkman and Okma, 1997). However, the 'pillarisation' of Dutch society began to weaken in the 1960s when state intervention became more pronounced as reflected in elements of universalism (Maarse, 1997). It is also at this time that home care was included in the new (social) insurance for exceptional medical risks and provided universal access to both health and social (home) care services (Coolen and Weekers, 1998: 50).

Japan

Although for many Westerners Japan is an enigma, its home care context shares much in common with Germany and the Netherlands. At its base, Japan has a communitarian, extended-family-based culture with veneration for the elderly. Although long-term care has until recently largely rested with the family, particularly women, for formal care this has meant that today universal coverage is widely accepted socially as a given. Moreover, during the last half-century traditional Japanese values have come into conflict with the infusion of a Western, largely American, individualistic culture, thus causing significant distress particularly among the older Japanese population.

Estonia

Since its independence in 1991, Estonia has adapted a Bismarckian-oriented health care system based on the principles of equality and solidarity. The health care system has undergone fundamental reforms, including the establishment of a compulsory health insurance, the decentralisation of the national health care administration, and the development of public health care (see Saks et al., 2003). The compulsory health insurance covers almost 95 per cent of Estonian residents and 80 to 90 per cent of the health care costs of insured people. The insurance guarantees almost all residents equal financial access to medical care. The home nursing service, which is also financed by the compulsory health insurance, was established in 2002. Domestic or social services are organised by the local governments. Access criteria are based on needs, and in the case of the elderly, the family situation. The local governments pay domestic services only for childless elderly. If children or grandchildren exist, the local governments decide whether and on what terms the senior citizen can receive domestic services.

Italy

The literature often characterises the Italian welfare state as 'conservative–corporatist' but the picture is more complex, especially in relation to home care where welfare arrangements are often 'rudimentary' (Tester, 1996). Informal care by women continues to be the norm, reflecting the strong role of the family in Italian society together with the perception of care as a family obligation (Convery and Cioni, 2001; Österle, 2001). Similar to Germany, at the formal level this expresses itself in the principle of subsidiarity. This is reflected in organisation of formal services where responsibilities are unclear and highly decentralised, public funding is patchy, provision is fragmented and the level of service provision is low (Polverini et al., 2004). In relation to health care, the principle of universalism was never fully implemented and co-payments for services remain high. The same applies to local social services and in home care where private funding solutions are fundamental. At the same time, health care as well as the local social services have seen the introduction of market mechanisms, which have produced a more mixed service provision but further complicated the boundary between the two services (Tester, 1996).

Sweden

Perhaps the clearest example of an egalitarian-type culture is Sweden, which is notable for the very early provision of medical care by the state dating back to the seventeenth century and an extensive range of social services 'from the cradle to the grave'. For instance, early on, towns and cities employed doctors to provide public health care and municipalities operated free hospitals, while in rural areas the central state paid physicians to provide basic care. State involvement in health care was consolidated in the middle of the nineteenth century with the creation of county councils which were chiefly responsible for health care. A considerable expansion of health services only occurred in the post-war period, however, paving the way for the universal health care system as we know it today. In the 1950s, social care services for the elderly were set up as a tax-based universal service organised by the local governments. The historical legacy of public involvement in health and social care is combined with the principle of equality, which is deeply embedded in Swedish society. People have a right to care regardless of income or where they live (Håkansson and Nordling, 1997). This right is part of a person's citizenship and not an individually earned entitlement as in the case of Germany and the Netherlands.

New Zealand

Although its political system compares most closely with that of the UK and its political culture retains many features of its Commonwealth heritage, like Sweden, New Zealand has a strong tradition of egalitarianism. This was clearly reflected in the Social Security Act of 1938, which committed an open-ended provision of health care to all citizens based on need. It is also demonstrated by the strong belief in the public consultation process and the view that office holders are holders of the public trust, not above it. New Zealand's egalitarian foundation is also illustrated by the 'tall poppy' belief that people who get too successful, wealthy or powerful must be cut back to size. For example, New Zealand politicians initially embraced the New Right market-centred philosophy in the 1980s and 1990s, but the public rejected attempts to restructure the health system in ways that were seen as destroying its egalitarian foundations. The result has been a series of rather bold attempts by governments of both parties to make major changes in society, only to pull back from more extreme and unpopular tactics once the public felt threatened and demanded a return to a more egalitarian system. Home care has not been high on the agenda in New Zealand, perhaps due in part to its relatively young population.

United Kingdom

In comparison to Sweden, the UK not only has had a much shorter history of public involvement in health and social care but its approach to collective action typically has been pragmatic and empirical rather than principled (Johnson and Cullen, 2000). This pattern helps to explain why after the Second World War a universal health service was introduced in what was traditionally a liberal state regime. The National Health Service (NHS), however, did not resolve the tension between *laissez-faire* liberalism and collectivism and as a result a rather generous entitlement philosophy has co-existed with rationed service provision (Moran, 1999). This has also meant that home (health) care for older people has been part of the NHS by default rather than design and has always co-existed with local, means-tested social care services. The health and social care divide has thus been a salient issue in as much as formal services have de facto been heavily complemented by informal care (Lewis, 2001). The fragmentation of home care contrasts with the fact that the principle of universalism together with a centralist political system makes for public expectations that health and social services be the same (or at least comparable) across the country.

United States

The United States is the prototype of an individualistic society.[5] Although individual rights are a consideration in all Western democracies, in the US rights have been elevated to a status of supremacy over collective interests. Moreover, by rights Americans mean 'negative' rights that require minimal government intervention and discount the notion of public goods, opting instead for a system where individuals largely fend for themselves. As a result, Americans are hesitant to sacrifice perceived individual needs for the common good. Moreover, when individual rights and the common good come into conflict, individual claims take precedence. Reinforcing the predominance of negative rights, US culture is also predisposed towards progress through technological means. The result has been an unrealistic dependence on technology to fix social problems at the expense of non-technological solutions. As a result, there has been extraordinary emphasis in the US on placing elderly people in institutional settings, particularly hospital-based ones where the best care is that which uses the most sophisticated new techniques. On the other hand, in the individualistic US informal home care support is minimal and citizens are expected to fend for themselves.

Home Care Statistics

One would expect these social and cultural variations among countries to be reflected in statistics on home care delivery and expenditures. However, one of the difficulties of analysing home care comparatively is that international statistics on home care are sparse. In part this is due to the diverse, informal and largely non-public sources of funding, which make it difficult to capture in one single figure how much is spent on home care. Also, because the organisation of home care is often highly decentralised, it is difficult to gather standardised figures across different localities let alone different countries. Not surprisingly, the statistics are often incomplete and in the main are not directly about home care. As a result, one usually can only extrapolate from trends in the more general category of long-term care or of institutionally-based care, for which more statistics are available, in order to get a sense of the degrees of de-institutionalisation in different countries. The question as to whether de-institutionalisation has been followed by the development of alternative formal home care services, however, remains unanswerable to a large degree.

The percentage of over 65 year-olds receiving formal home care services in Table 1.3 offers a more direct indication of the relative size of home care services. In the Netherlands, Sweden and the US more than 11 per cent of older people receive formal help at home. With 16 per cent, the US is a clear outlier. This figure, however, probably does not reflect a generosity on the part of government but rather the vigorous marketing of many private, long-term care insurance plans. In the other countries, between 9.6 per cent (in Germany) and 3 per cent (in Italy) of older people receive formal home care services. Although in all countries only a minority of older people receive formal help, the variation among countries is clear. However, this might disguise the fact that many older people living in their own home rely on informal care from female relatives. With the exception of Italy and Japan, in all countries the percentage of older people receiving formal home care is greater than the percentage living in institutions. This highlights the importance of home care for older people. It is at home where the majority of older people reside.

Table 1.3 Percentage of population aged 65 and over in different care settings

	In institutions	Receiving formal help at home
Estonia*		
Germany	6.8	9.6
Italy	3.9	3.0
Japan	6.0	5.0
Netherlands	8.8	12.0
Sweden	8.7	11.2
UK	5.1	5.5
US	5.7	16.0

Note: *2.6% Tallinn (capital), 1.5% Tartu (domestic service only), taken from Saks et al. (2003).

Source: Jacobzone (1999).

Despite the inconclusive trends in the provision of institutionally-based care, the spending on other types of services for the elderly and disabled has increased significantly. Table 1.4 lists per capita public expenditure on day care, rehabilitation, home help services and other services in kind. With the exception of New Zealand and the US, in all of our countries public spending increased between 1983 and 1998, ranging from twofold or less in Italy, the Netherlands and the UK to over fourfold in Japan. Sweden continues to spend the highest per capita by far and jumped by almost fourfold during these years.

Preliminary data on expenditures for home care across these countries

Table 1.4 Per capita public expenditure on services for the elderly and disabled (in US dollars)

	1983[1]	1988	1993	1998[2]	Rates of increase
Germany	44	62	111	166	3.8
Italy	21	33	44	42	2.0
Japan	17	24	44	73	4.3
Netherlands	72	77	98	102	1.4
New Zealand	4	4	4	1	n/a
Sweden	202	289	571	791	3.9
UK	54	76	114	116	2.1
US	1	13	15	12	n/a

Notes:
1. This is the first year for which figures are available.
2. The figures refer to 1997, the most recent year for which figures are available.

Source: OECD (2001b).

demonstrate considerable variation as well. Table 1.5 shows total expenditure on home care as a percentage of GDP ranging from 0.02 per cent in Japan to 0.82 per cent in Sweden. Similar differences are apparent in the public and private distributions for home care and the comparison with spending on institutional care, which in most countries represents multiples of home care spending. Again the limits of the data must be reiterated, however, because they are unlikely to reflect the costs of informal home care supplied by family and friends. These issues will be analysed in more detail in the substantive chapters on formal and informal care givers.

The analysis of available statistics has given a preliminary overview of home care in our countries. In terms of both funding and provision, formalised home care is marginal in these countries, more so in some than in others. At the same time there is no clear evidence for systematic moves away from institutionally-based care. Nevertheless, more public money is being spent on alternative services for older people, such as day centres and home helps. Most importantly, the analysis of the statistics highlights the need to locate home care in the different health and social welfare systems in which it is embedded. While the delivery, funding and rules of home care will be examined in detail in the following chapters, it is useful here to provide a quick review of the complicated nature of governing this amorphous and inclusive area of home care.

Table 1.5 Expenditures on long-term care as a percentage of GDP, 2000

	Public expenditure		Private expenditure		Total expenditure		
	Home	Institutional	Home	Institutional	Home	Institutional	Total
Germany	0.43	0.52	0.04	0.36	0.47	0.88	1.35
Japan	0.02	0.69	0.00	0.07	0.02	0.76	0.78
Netherlands	0.56	0.75	0.05	0.08	0.61	0.83	1.44
New Zealand	0.11	0.34	0.01	0.22	0.12	0.56	0.68
Sweden	0.78	1.96	0.04	0.10	0.82	2.07	2.89
UK	0.32	0.58	0.09	0.38	0.41	0.96	1.37
US	0.17	0.58	0.16	0.39	0.33	0.96	1.29

Source: OECD (2004).

DEVELOPMENTS IN HOME CARE GOVERNANCE

Thus far we have outlined what we mean by home care and home care governance and have introduced the need to analyse variation across countries. We now turn our attention to the dynamics of home care brought about by demographic, social and economic changes. Although there are many demographic factors impacting on home care, such as increased mobility and immigration, the single most important and ubiquitous is the ageing of populations. Similarly, while social changes are many, the individualisation and liberalisation of societies have led women especially to articulate their needs in different ways, which have considerable ramifications for home care. Finally, often pulling in opposite directions, economic constraints on the one hand mean that traditional home care givers are forced into the workplace to make ends meet and on the other mean that public resources have become more scarce, thus squeezing traditional welfare systems. Because of their importance for the governance of home care, we now look at each of these sets of dynamics in turn.

The Problem of Ageing Populations

There is no doubt that a major reason forcing all countries to intensify the need to address home care and to engage more actively in governing home care is the ageing of their populations. As illustrated in Table 1.6, all countries will experience significant ageing of their populations over the next 30 years. Although the ageing process is taking place earlier and more rapidly in some countries, all are expected to experience the ageing process that began in the

Table 1.6 Percentage of population aged 65 and over

	1960	1980	1990	2000	2020	2030	2040
Estonia	–	–	15.5	–	19–20	–	
Germany	10.8	15.5	15.3	16.8	21.7	25.8	27.6
Italy	10.5	13.2	14.9	17.6	19.4	21.9	24.2
Japan	5.7	9.1	12.1	16.7	20.9	21.0	22.7
Netherlands	9.0	11.5	12.8	13.6	18.9	23.0	24.8
New Zealand	8.7	9.7	11.1	11.7	15.3	19.4	21.9
Sweden	11.8	16.3	17.8	17.8	20.8	21.7	22.5
UK	11.7	15.0	15.7	15.7	16.3	19.2	20.4
US	9.2	11.2	12.4	12.3	16.2	19.5	19.8

Sources: OECD (1988); for Estonia: Saks et al. (2003).

1970s and is now accelerating particularly in the non-European countries, which currently have younger populations. The primary cause of the ageing of Western societies is the precipitous decline in fertility rates, which has naturally increased the proportion of elderly. This trend is exaggerated, however, because the sharp upturn in birth rates after the Second World War produced a bloated age cohort in the 'baby boom' generation, the first wave of which is now approaching retirement age. Even if life expectancy is not lengthened over the coming decades, this upsurge of ageing baby boomers combined with low fertility rates guarantees an increasing proportion of elderly candidates for home care.

A complicating factor is increased life expectancy. In the 30 years between 1950 and 1980, life expectancy at birth on average increased by 8.5 years for females and 6.0 years for males. These sizeable gains result from improved social conditions, health habits, and the new capacities of medicine to reduce infant mortality and extend the life span. Ironically, although our advances in medical science can significantly extend the lives of the older patients, often the lives saved are at a lower quality of life and a frailty which requires even more social care over extended periods of time. According to Eurostat, these big rises in the elderly will have 'profound consequences' for social protection systems: 'EU-wide, the share of the elderly in the total population is expected to rise from 21% now to around 34% by 2050. Those 80+ are predicted to rise from 4% of today's population to some 10%. By 2050, 37 million people are expected to be octogenarians+' (Eurostat News Release, 1999).

These ageing trends are accompanied by two changes in the population structure that are critical for home care. First, within the overall trends towards older populations is the ageing of these elderly populations themselves. At present the most rapidly growing segment of the elderly population is the cohort aged 80 and over, which currently represents the age group with the greatest need for home care. As illustrated in Table 1.7, by 2050 this proportion is expected to climb to over 30 per cent across Western countries. The second trend relates to the sex composition of the elderly population. As

Table 1.7 Estimated age structure of proportion of the population aged 65 and over, OECD

	1980	1990	2000	2010	2020	2030	2040	2050
65–69	34	32	31	32	31	31	27	26
70–79	48	46	48	44	46	46	47	43
80/over	18	22	22	24	22	24	26	31

Source: OECD (1988: 23).

a result of their longer life expectancy, women outnumber men by significant margins in the elderly age cohorts. Furthermore, the sex imbalance increases with age, meaning that as the very elderly cohort expands, the proportion of elderly women will increase. This is particularly crucial for home care, since traditionally women have borne the brunt of home care but now also represent the largest group of users.

Social Trends

Reinforcing these demographic shifts are the substantial social transformations in modern societies that accompany the individualisation and liberalisation of traditional values. Just at the time when there is an increased need for long-term care giving, social changes have begun to undermine traditional, largely informal and family-based care, mechanisms of care for the elderly. The decline in the extended family and more recently the nuclear family, increased mobility, and trends towards secularisation have undermined traditional support systems and put added pressures on governments to fill the gap.

Moreover, in combination with the economic constraints discussed below, social movements towards equality for women have encouraged more women today to seek fulfilment through a career, with the result in many countries of reducing the supply of informal, unpaid care givers. Within this new cultural milieu, women are less likely than in the past to be willing or able to forgo paid employment to serve as a care giver. Table 1.8 shows the magnitude of the increase of women in the workplace in our countries. Although women continue to provide significant levels of long-term care for family members, coverage is saturated and as a proportion will continue to decrease just when

Table 1.8 Labour force participation rates of women, 1973–2003

	1973	1979	1983	1993	1999	2003
Germany	50.3	52.2	52.5	61.8	63.0	64.5
Italy	33.7	38.7	40.3	43.3	45.5	48.3
Japan	54.0	54.7	57.2	61.8	59.5	59.7
Netherlands	29.2	33.4	40.3	56.0	64.4	68.4
New Zealand	39.2	45.0	45.7	63.2	67.4	69.3
Sweden	62.6	72.8	76.6	75.8	76.0	76.9
UK	53.2	58.0	57.2	65.3	68.4	69.2
US	51.1	58.7	61.9	69.0	70.7	69.7

Sources: 1973–93, OECD (1996); 1999–2003, OECD (2004).

the need for home care for the elderly deepens. As a result, the demands for formal long-term care services will increase to meet expanding need, and such services will depend increasingly on public funds. Those countries without adequate planning and funding infrastructures for long-term care are especially vulnerable to severe problems in this regard.

Economic Trends

All Western countries are experiencing difficulties in meeting expanding demands for long-term care and other services as jobs are lost in globalisation, their populations age, and public resources become scarcer. Home care is seen by some observers as a way to square the circle among these demographic and cost pressures (Duff, 2001). This is based on the presumption that care in the home is much cheaper than care provided in labour-intensive hospitals and nursing homes. Substituting care in the home for institutionally-based care is also said to be better for older people, because home-based settings make it easier to combine formal with informal care arrangements.

This shift in priorities also reflects the more critical attitudes towards the institutionalisation of older people that emerged in the 1970s (Jenson and Jacobzone, 2000). Substitution policies refer to a set of policies that aim to replace institutionally-based care with care in the home and related settings. De-institutionalisation driven by either financial or humanitarian motivations, however, without sufficient development of non-institutional settings can result in additional demands on women as informal carers (ibid.). When assessing the provision of home care it is important to look at how services are organised and who provides these services. Both aspects give an indication of the degree to which home care is integrated into health and social care systems and influences the level of service provision.

The Dynamics of Home Care Governance

These three sets of factors – demographic, social and economic – have combined to create a dynamic and fluid environment for home care, especially in terms of finance. The ways in which home care is funded are significant in two respects. Security of funding, together with the relative level of (public) funding, are important factors shaping the provision of home care services. Funding arrangements also give an indication of the extent to which home care is an integral part of a health and/or social welfare system. The funding sources of formal home care can range from taxes and social insurance contributions to out-of-pocket payments and private insurance. The first two make for secure if not necessarily sufficient funding, whereas out-of-pocket payments are the least reliable and equitable sources of funding. The funding of home care is typically highly mixed and a substantial amount of home care is funded out of out-of-pocket payments. Moreover, public funding is often not secure and hardly sufficient and has to be supplemented by out-of-pocket payments.

Furthermore, often the level of service provision is very basic and involves a diverse range of providers. As a result, the emphasis on welfare mix competes with the policy goals of integrating services across different providers and reducing the divide between health and social care. Moreover, the discussion thus far has focused only on formal home care, that is, the care provided by paid staff with formal training/qualifications. Home care becomes even more complicated when it is realised that the majority of home care has traditionally been and still is provided by family and friends, that is, informal unpaid carers. Tester (1996), in her comparison of community care in a number of European countries and the US, estimates that informal carers provide 75 to 80 per cent of care, a figure largely borne out across many studies. With cost containment in health care and inadequate resources to develop home care services, the burden on informal carers actually has increased in recent years. Substitution policies also mean that home care services are regularly targeted at highly dependent older people who would otherwise require institutional care.

We would expect variation across countries regarding the importance of informal care in relation to underlying cultural assumptions about the role of the family (and women in particular) in care giving. In those countries where family bonds and collectivist values are traditionally strong, care-giving responsibilities of families should be more extensive with the opposite applying to countries where values of individual independence dominate. In the latter countries it will be more accepted that care giving be in the hands of paid professionals or at least that they complement informal care. With home care now on the political agenda of many countries, interest in informal care has broadened. Home is where the vast majority of older people live with their spouses and partners, and home is also one of the places where older people meet with friends and family. The spatial interface of personal relationships and home care facilitates the provision of informal care. Not surprisingly, most home care policies have acknowledged the importance of informal care. From a comparative perspective, the interesting question is what this acknowledgement means in practice and how governance defines the interface between formal and informal care.

Here a number of considerations come into play. In times of resource constraints it seems inevitable that home care systems will continue to rely on informal care. Compared to formal care this is the less costly option, but only if the costs associated with informal care (such as lost income and pension entitlements) are ignored (Jacobszone, 1999). Another consideration is that the expansion of formal care might lead to the reduction of the provision of informal care and even create additional demands for formal care (Jamieson, 1996). This can be either a desirable or an undesirable policy outcome, although studies indicate that substitution is not necessarily straightforward either way. For moderately disabled older people, home-based care is likely to be the best (and most efficient) option. In contrast, for severely disabled older people, institutional care is more appropriate (Jacobzone, 1999). If anything this suggests that substitution needs to be tailored to the particular circumstances of individuals (Low et al., 2000). Moreover, even in countries with relatively high levels of publicly-funded formal care, families, primarily women, continue to play a significant role as informal carers. Nevertheless, the pool of informal carers is ultimately limited and home care cannot continue to function without formal care (Twigg, 1996).

Policies on the informal aspects of home care pick and mix considerations about the interface between the formal and the informal in distinct ways. In turn they are shaped by cultural assumptions about the role of the family in care giving. At the same time, it is interesting that in recent years many countries have experimented in one way or another with a more explicit integration of informal care into the formal health system. Twigg (ibid.) has developed a typology for understanding the range of relationships that exist between welfare agencies and informal carers. She distinguishes the following types: carers as resources where carers are taken for granted; carers as co-workers where carers are treated instrumentally to ensure the continuation of their caring activities; carers as co-clients where agencies are concerned with the needs of carers in their own right; and superseded carers where agencies aim to replace carers with paid formal care staff.

Home care therefore is full of contradictions. Home care is varied and diverse yet it is an indispensable need across all countries. Home care is hardly visible in international statistics yet it is central to the health and well-being of an increasing number of people. Home care funding and provision is often fragmented, yet home care is of increasing importance on the policy agenda of many countries. These are some of the salient contradictions in home care. An interesting question is how are recent policy trends and developments altering home care in response to the demographic, social and economic pressures discussed earlier?

The provision of home care services is diverse and this diversity means a greater number and wider range of providers. This requires greater coordination but at the same time makes coordination and ultimately the integration into the health system more difficult. Problems of coordination can be exacerbated by a sharp divide between different types of care (for example, health and social care in the UK), the absence of national legislation (as in the case of the US) or highly decentralised governance structures (as in the case of Sweden). Also it is likely that diversity of provision does not necessarily translate into adequate levels of provision. This gives credence to the more general tenet that in times of cost containment increased diversity of provision often coincides with a targeting of services to those in greatest need or to those without any other means.

Regardless of the policy trends in the provision and funding of services, home care remains overwhelmingly informal women's work. In comparison to formal home care, informal women's work continues to be cheap and readily available in most countries. Irrespective of differences among political systems and cultural attitudes towards the role of women, however, the majority of countries have started to acknowledge the centrality of informal care. This takes different forms, ranging from the gender-blindness of liberal welfare traditions (such as in the US) and gender-specific expectations in traditionally male-dominated collectivist societies (such as in Japan), to the ideology of welfare society (such as in the UK and Sweden), the revival of subsidiarity (in Germany), and payments of carers (such as in Germany and the Netherlands). What has changed is that the marginality of informal home care has come more sharply into focus and the demographic, social and economic pressures for more far-reaching and meaningful governance of this area has intensified.

CHAPTERS THAT FOLLOW

Chapter 2 explains the foundations of the analytical framework and identifies its innovative features. It defines home care governance as consisting of a range of issues around the organisation of formal care services, the identification of informal care, the definition of the professional territories of care workers and the terms under which care users are included in home care. The chapter explores different approaches of analysing home care governance and presents the social care and the public policy literature as two complementary theoretical perspectives. It uses the questions raised by each body of literature to build a more inclusive conceptual framework for analysing and explaining home care governance across countries. Chapter 3 extends this introduction to the empirical chapters by demonstrating how to conceptualise the context of home care governance, particularly the institutions and ideas that are its key components. It thus provides a systematic analysis of the contexts of home care governance across our countries.

Chapter 4 focuses on formal care services and analyses governance arrangements as related to their organisation. Such governance arrangements are becoming higher on the political agenda in many countries, reflecting the perception that the needs of an increasingly older, and often politically astute, population are confronted with falling resources of informal care and constrained financial resources. Governance is therefore caught between expanding and containing formal care services, and the chapter analyses which direction governance is taking across different countries and how this can be explained. Prevailing ideas about gender relations in the labour market are particularly important here, and are also reflected in the dominant modes of funding and providing formal care services. This chapter analyses governing arrangements in relation to formal care services in terms of the relative degrees of integration and fragmentation, looking at governing through provision, funding and rules. From a cross-country comparative perspective, the chapter also explores which types of ideas and institutions as the context of home care governance provide more or less favourable conditions for relatively integrated governing arrangements.

Chapter 5 turns attention to informal home care and looks at the changing boundaries between formal and informal care. The focus is on the integration of informal care in the overall provision of care embedded in different institutional settings and its relationship to daily caring activities on a micro level, as well as the consequences for the relations between men and women, social classes and ethnic groups in society. The new approaches concern the distribution of care activities between the family or informal sector and different sectors located in the public sphere, the ascription of societal and family responsibilities and the distribution of costs. The new regulations extend mechanisms of governance to the area of informal care within the family framework and establish thus a mode of coordination which includes the state, market, associations and family. The chapter also examines employment contracts regarding wages and regulations on the labour market and the control of the caring activities.

Chapter 6 turns attention to the governance arrangements relating to care workers in home care. The formalisation of care arrangements, especially as it occurs under tight financial constraints, has raised issues about the boundaries of paid, qualified care workers in relation to informal carers and about the level of training required for different care tasks. This leads to conflicts between professional and economic interests, and this chapter examines what shape this conflict takes in different contexts and how this in turn influences governing arrangements concerned with defining professional territory across countries. Here the analysis looks at a number of factors, including prevalent ideas about gender relations and how they influence ideas about the right size and composition of professional territories in home care, the diversity of care workers as a group and how this relates to different degrees of plasticity of care, the relative existence of alliances between care workers and other actors, and the relative degree of institutional integration of funding and provision arrangements, and its importance as an incentive for developing home care as a territory for paid and qualified care workers. The discussion of the relative health and social care occupational orientation of care workers suggests that social care orientations dominate and that this is also closely associated with a relatively weak institutionalisation of care work as an occupational activity. The variations among countries found in Chapter 6 point to important country-specific combinations of dissimilar aspects of the institutional context of home care governance, in particular the relative support for female employment and for formal care services, respectively.

Using the notions of consumer and citizen, Chapter 7 analyses the consequences of processes of individualisation in society by contrasting the concepts of consumerism and social and citizenship rights. As individual actors, the care recipients themselves are examined according to their opportunities to determine their individual care arrangement. The analysis looks at elements of the institutional contexts which affect the actions of the individual and collective actors such as the definition and implementation of social rights, related modes of funding via taxes or social insurance contributions and eligibility criteria, as well as features of service organisation such as diversification and offers and genuine choice. Significantly, both aspects are strongly embedded in specific mixes of different modes of coordination of home care, that is, mainly state regulations and market. The chapter finds that with the introduction of the long-term care insurance, the role of the users has been changed within a newly regulated care infrastructure oriented towards market principles.

The concluding chapter returns to the comparative context of governing home care. It attempts to categorise governing arrangements regarding the funding, delivery and rules of home care, and the formal/informal mix based on the factors identified in the substantive chapters as the most crucial. It summarises the findings concerning the logics and instruments of home care governance introduced in Chapter 1 and reviews what we have learned about patterns and differences in home care governance across these countries. This chapter also analyses to what extent these disparate countries are dealing with the challenges raised by home care. How well are the many challenges of the twenty-first century being translated into workable governance arrangements and how do the variable policies reflect the institutional and value differences across these countries? Finally, are governance initiatives across these countries leading to a policy convergence in home care in the light of the trends noted above or continued divergence?

NOTES

1. The concept of governance and its implications for the study of home care are extended in Chapters 2 and 3, which map out the ideas and institutions that form the context of the governance of home care in our countries.

2. This chapter presents broader more general political, cultural and historical contexts, while Chapter 3 defines these contexts in considerably more detail.
3. We have not expanded our analysis to include developing nations because we felt this would inextricably complicate the analysis. Although inclusion of a sample of such countries might be interesting, we believe that this more focused analysis is more fruitful at this stage.
4. In relation to the UK, the political devolution since the late 1990s has meant that home care policies in the four countries of the UK have started to diverge. The analysis presented in this book is primarily about policies as they apply to England. As the focus of the analysis is on comparing between (rather than within) countries, the analysis refers to the UK throughout the book.
5. The closest other being Australia.

2. Analysing home care governance: bringing together different conceptual perspectives

The first chapter began by discussing the specificities of home care and pointed to the fact that home care cuts across different boundaries, especially the boundaries between the public and the private, and between the micro and the macro levels. The chapter then introduced the concept of governance, understood as a combination of different modes of coordination needed to capture the complex nature of home care. On this basis, it presented an analytical framework for studying home care governance from a comparative perspective. The aim of the present chapter is twofold: to explain the source of the analytical framework and, by doing this, to identify its innovative features. This discussion also provides a basis for discussing the contribution of the analysis presented in the following chapters to the existing literature.

The aim of the analysis presented in this book is twofold: first, to systematically map out the governance of home care in relation to a number of areas of governing across our nine countries and, second, to explore the ways in which institutions and ideas (and the interplay between them) shape governing arrangements. This chapter first introduces the notion of governance and discusses how the notion of governance applies to the area of home care. Against this background, it then explores different approaches to analysing home care governance and presents the social care and the public policy literature as two different yet complementary theoretical perspectives.

CONCEPTUALISING THE GOVERNANCE OF HOME CARE

As Chapter 1 suggests, home care is an area that cuts across many boundaries, especially between the formal and informal and between the public and private. The state is a relative latecomer in relation to home care, and the high degree of societal embeddedness of home care makes for complex forms of coordination. To capture this complexity we use the concept of governance. The concept has become a widely used analytical tool in public policy research (for an overview, see Kooiman, 2000 and Kjær, 2004). The central focus is the capacity of governments to exert influence in the context of nation states. According to Kooiman and van Vliet (1993), governments no longer have the capacity to determine social developments in more complex, dynamic and diverse societies. Instead, government increasingly engages in co-regulation, whereby boundaries between government and society and between public and private sectors are becoming blurred. The concept of governance therefore focuses on new ways of coordination that go beyond the state and include the market as well as networks as alternative ways of steering.

In contrast, the concept of governance is used much less in social policy research (for exceptions, see Newman, 2001; Daly, 2003). In her discussion of how to transfer of the concept of governance to social policy, Daly highlights the ability of the concept to connect state/civil society activities of co-ordination across different (local, regional and national) levels. Furthermore, the concept of governance focuses on policy development, which enables the explanation of the how and why of welfare state reform. Daly is critical of the emphasis on procedures rather than the content of policies, which in her view neglects the relationship between policy and societal developments.

Our analysis of the governance of home care brings together both strands of research to provide a more integrated framework of analysis. Research on social care defines the characteristics of the area of home care as an area of governance and focuses on the content of policies, thereby revealing its embeddedness in society, while public policy research provides the tools for analysing policy development and procedures. Before doing this, however, we first present our definition of governance. As Newman (2001) critically observes, the concept of governance is a widely used but often elusive analytical tool. Governance is an umbrella concept that lacks a coherent body of theory and that is applied in a wide variety of contexts.

Table 2.1 presents home care governance as consisting of distinct sets of logics and instruments which have to be adapted to the decisive characteristics of the area of home care. The logics of home care governance describe the broader ideas underlying its different types. The typology used here follows Streeck and Schmitter's (1985; similarly in relation to social care, see Anttonen et al., 2003) now classical distinction between state, associations, the market and the family (originally referred to as the community). This range of logics of home care governance also echoes the different emphases of the two literatures. While the public policy perspective often focuses on the state and its importance relative to the competing logics of *associations* and the *market*, the social care perspective takes the logic of the *family* and its relationship to the (welfare) state as the starting-point. In the specific case of home care the logic of associations, with its concern for inter-organisational dynamics, specifically includes professionalism, reflecting the importance of professions in home care. Table 2.1 describes the logics of home care governance as ideal

Table 2.1 Logics and instruments of home care governance (2)

Logics of home care governance	Instruments of home care governance		
	Delivery	Funding	Rules
State	Formal/public	Public (through taxes, social insurance)	Hierarchy; through command-and-control rules such as laws and regulations
Associations	Formal/private, non-profit	Private donations, membership/professional dues	Norms; through negotiations and ethic codes
Market	Formal/private, for-profit	Private insurance, out-of pocket payments	Profit seeking; through competition
Family	Informal/private	Indirect transfers (through family income)	Moral/personal obligation; through emotional/social relations

types, whereas the thematic analysis in the following chapters presents a more dynamic picture of changes within the area. Here, Beck Jørgensen and Vrangbæk (2004) suggest distinguishing between three sets of dynamics: changes *within* individual ideal types (for example, in respect to their characteristic features), changes *between* different ideal types (for example, concerning their relative importance), and the existence of *hybrids*, which combine elements of different ideal types.

The instruments of home care governance in turn help to further specify what these logics mean in practice and also suggest that logics vary among instruments. Here, delivery, funding and rules describe distinct sets of instruments of coordinating home care which are also associated with different degrees of involvement or intervention in the case of the logic of the state (see Alber, 1995; Howlett and Ramesh, 2003). In relation to rules, Table 2.1 refers to both the key principle and associated mechanism of governing. Again, the range of instruments of home care governance reflects the different emphases of the two literatures. The social care perspective is particularly concerned with delivery and to a lesser extent funding and the content of rules, whereas the public policy perspective focuses especially on governance through rule setting.

So what are the characteristics of the different types of home care governance? The logic of the state is typically associated with formal and public delivery, and funding following the logic of the state occurs either through taxes or social insurance contributions. Following the principle of hierarchy, rules take the form of command-and-control rules. This contrasts with the logic of associations, where delivery, while still formal, is private, non-profit, and where private funding in the form of donations and membership/professional dues dominates. In this logic, rules are based on the principle of norms and often take the form of negotiations and ethic codes. The logic of the market is related to delivery that is formal and private but for-profit, and private funding in the form of donations and professional dues is prevalent. Rules follow the principle of profit seeking and competition among autonomous actors is the key mechanism of this logic of governance. Finally, the logic of the family is distinct, in that delivery is private but informal, and funding relies on indirect transfers from the family income. Rules are derived from the principle of moral/personal obligation, and tend to take the form of emotional/social relations.

The governance of home care has been conceptualised as different logics and instruments related to the coordination of home care activities. Against this background, the remainder of the chapter explores in more detail different approaches to analysing home care governance. The feminist social care approach is dominant in the field and is most concerned with the (gendered) nature of home care on the one hand, and how the formal institutions of the welfare state, especially the social institutions of the family together with ideas around gender, shape the governance of home care on the other. In contrast, the public policy literature has been marginal to the field to date but makes a number of contributions to the comparative study of home care governance. First, with its focus on the political system and policy subsystems, this literature introduces a different set of formal institutions from the social care literature. Second, the literature is more extensively concerned with the dynamics of governing. This reflects greater interest as compared with the social care literature, in the interplay between institutions and ideas, especially in relation to the process of policy development.

THE CONCEPT OF SOCIAL CARE AND ITS CONTRIBUTION TO ANALYSING HOME CARE GOVERNANCE

The concept of social care is reviewed here to show its contribution to the analysis of home care governance. It is argued that the concept and its implications are important in respect to three issues. First, the concept of social care clarifies the significant dimensions for an analysis of the activity of social care, its societal embeddedness and its gender and social implications. Second, the concepts used for the analysis of social care point to the central issues of social care (and its governance) and how governance issues also become a part of public debate and public policy. Third, cross-country studies clarify the fundamental dimensions for the comparison of different approaches to social care governance. The literature reveals social care as a multifaceted activity which cuts across traditional boundaries, especially between the public and private spheres as well as its implications for gender relations and governance approaches in this area. While on a conceptual level the process of policy development is a neglected area, the concept of social care may be used for the analysis of the framing of policies, the underlying values and institutional regulations.

Dimensions of Social Care

In the 1980s, the concept of social care began to be developed within British and Scandinavian feminist research for the analysis of until then a neglected area in scientific research, which was viewed as decisive for the societal position of women (see Finch and Groves, 1983; Hernes, 1984, 1987a, b; Waerness, 1984). Initially, the research aimed at revealing the widespread care activities of women, key features of the day-to-day practice on the micro level, and their relationship to the disadvantageous situation of women in society in both the public and private spheres. In the UK, the focus of the first type of research was on unpaid care work carried out by women within the family framework, while in the northern countries the entry of women into paid employment was taken as a starting-point for the analysis of paid care work and its implications for the position of women in society.

The dichotomy between paid and unpaid care in predominant theoretical conceptions and empirical research was criticised by Ungerson (1990), leading to the development of approaches for a more comprehensive concept of social care. Characteristic dimensions of social care work such as the identity of the carer and the care receiver, the relationship of carer and care receiver, the setting or social domain of care work, and the nature of care and the economic character of the care relationship were proposed by Thomas (1993) as guidelines for a comprehensive empirical research that cuts across boundaries. The inclusion of non-kin forms of home care (for example, care work by domestic servants) proved that social care was a gendered issue, and raised the question of relationship to class and ethnicity in society (Graham, 1991; Hochschild, 2000; Hondagneu-Sotelo, 2000). Even from the perspective of the care receivers, patterns of informal care giving and access to formal services can be detected which are related to gender, ethnicity and social position (Tester, 1996; Glendinning, 1998; Blinkert and Klie, 1999). The relationship of gender, social class and ethnicity varies among countries dependent on the social care approach selected by the individual welfare state (Anttonen and Sipilä, 1996; Theobald, 2003, 2005).

Early gender-sensitive research on social care was concentrated on the micro level (the context and content of daily care activities and its implications). In contrast, welfare mix and social care approaches define fundamental dimensions of social care delivery on a macro level. The welfare-mix approach of Evers and his colleagues proceeds on the assumption that different areas of care provision (the state, the market, the voluntary sector and the family) are evident in all European countries, though the countries differ in regard to the significance and scope of the areas as well as their organisation and funding (Evers and Wintersberger, 1990; Evers and Svetlik, 1993). Evers and his colleagues assign different underlying rationales to the areas. Universalistic orientations predominate at the state level, while values of instrumentalism and choice are uppermost in the market. In the family and in the voluntary sector, norms and traditions of personal obligation and linkage are prevalent.

Within the social care model approach, different dimensions of social care delivery and their implications are used to assign countries to different models. Anttonen and Sipilä (1996) defined the dimensions of 'way of organising' and 'volume of care services' as criteria for their model. In the further refinement of the social care model approach, the dimensions were extended to include those such as the area of provision of care and funding (Szebehely, 1999a,b), the implications of different modes of care delivery for the care receivers and carers (Sipilä and Anttonen, 1999; Stark and Regner, 2002), and the regulation of access to services (Anttonen et al., 2003).

In contrast, Daly and Lewis (1998) combine in their approach both micro- and macro-level analysis. They define the concept of social care as multi-faceted with three dimensions that cross boundaries between the public and private spheres and are located on both the macro and the micro levels. The first dimension emphasises care as labour, and analyses the nature and conditions of care work within the family framework and in the labour market, and its interplay and relationship to care policies on the macro level. The second dimension views care within a normative framework of obligations and responsibilities. Here the focus is on the social relationships in caring activities and the definition of individual, familial and societal responsibility on both levels. The third dimension considers the sharing of financial and emotional costs of the care activity in daily care work and regulated within social care policies.

Daly and Lewis (1998) view the macro and micro levels as interwoven. They argue that the restructured division of labour, responsibility and costs among state, market, family and civil society during the 1990s within the newly developed care policies brought about new distributions and conditions of care work on the macro level and identities of formal and informal carers on the micro level. The way in which family members take over the responsibility of care has been revealed to be a matter of negotiation where the definition of family responsibility and the availability of services is considered. Family responsibilities do not operate by way of substantive fixed rules but are acknowledged as procedural guidelines that indicate how to take over responsibilities and work out an appropriate level of help to relatives (Finch, 1989; Finch and Mason, 1991, 1993).

In summary, the concept of social care reveals care as an activity which covers different areas, institutional settings, relations and norms, and crosses conventional boundaries such as private/public, paid/unpaid, formal/informal and micro/macro levels. The detailed insights into the substantive dimensions of social care offer a basis for identifying the characteristic features of home care as a field of governance and the relationships between the dimensions. It also shows the key role of gender and the implications of the activity of social care for gender and further social relations. Despite the neglect of a detailed analysis of the process of policy development, the dimensions provide indications on the key substantive dimensions for the analysis of such processes, for example, what issues are involved in the societal arrangements of social care, what actors or areas should be considered and what norms and ideas are related to specific areas and actors.

Care as a Public Good: The Issue of Rights and Settlements

Since the 1990s, the expected 'caring deficit' (Hochschild, 1995) due to demographic changes and the increasing female labour market participation has fostered a political debate about the adequate societal regulations and the needs, rights and responsibilities of the care dependant and the care provider. Daly (2002) distinguishes care as a public policy good through the issue of regulations and settlements on social care which are manifested in public policies, and care as a social good, that is, the issue of care as an activity related to norms and social relations in society. She argues that the high degree of political activity during the 1990s may be taken as an indicator of the rising public interest and settlements in this area. The introduction of welfare state regulations around social care involves the establishment of a bureaucracy as a set of rules and procedures. The regulations attached to the benefits and services reflect the assumptions about the obligations and tasks of the families and the society as well as men and women in care provision (Leira and Saraceno, 2003).

Referring to the different perspectives of care as a public and as a social good, Daly (2002) describes two strands in the debate on social care. One strand that has been developed in feminist welfare state research views care activities embedded in society and their implication for gender relations (see section above). The second strand discusses how social policy approaches manage the demand and supply of care, or how the interests of both the care receivers and the carers can be met. This latter analysis of care provision is concerned with the issues concerning the adequate type of provision and funding and allocation principles. Different types of care provision such as cash and in-kind benefits, leave arrangements, services or vouchers, have been offered that aim at providing the care receivers and informal carers with time, money and services (Daly, 2000; Bettio and Plantenga, 2004).

Public policies on care are concerned not only with the definition of the type of support but also with the range and level of collective funding and rules of accessibility. Pacolet et al. (2000) summarise two basic types of funding long-term care that can be found in elderly care approaches in European countries. In the Nordic countries and the UK, funding principles via taxes within the health and social care schemes are prevalent. In some Continental European countries, separate mainly social insurance-based funding schemes have been introduced in the 1990s. Neither type of funding covers all costs of long-term care and despite country differences a care hierarchy is evident. Care strongly connected to nursing care is more often covered as household or social services (ibid.). Despite welfare state differences, in most countries there is a moral obligation for relatives to take responsibility for the care of their elderly relatives and/or to take financial responsibility for the services. The right to be cared for is still an incomplete social right (Knijn and Kremer, 1997; Leira and Saraceno, 2003).

Furthermore, Österle (2001) and Anttonen et al. (2003a) analyse the accessibility of different types of care provision. While Anttonen et al. use the terms 'individualisation' and 'universalisation' as two basic principles regulating the access to care services and benefits, Österle assesses norms related to the level of support using the terms 'equity' or 'fairness'. Individualisation relates to whether and to what extent publicly funded social care services are allocated on the basis of the family status or on the needs of the individual. Universalisation refers to whether and to what extent the allocation of social care is selective, typically based on means-tested procedures or universal availability. On the basis of their approach, Anttonen et al. assign specific care services to certain points in the two dimensions and use them as criteria for the quality of services.

Österle distinguishes three levels of allocated resources that are related to different social policy goals: the first, 'guaranteeing minimum standards', aims at preventing the risk of poverty in the case of care dependency and provides only a minimum level of economic resources or services; the second, 'supporting living standards', grants a level of economic resources or services that prevent the elderly or the informal carers from large drops in their individual living situation; and the third, 'reducing inequality', relates the situation of the individual care receiver or informal carer to the average situation in a society. Here the key issues are the redistribution between the healthy and those in need, for example, through the definition of tax- or insurance-based coverage of the costs or between the wealthier and poorest people in society through the introduction of earnings-related co-payments.

In their overview of the development of social care research, Daly and Rake (2003) criticised this strand of research because of its tendency to focus on key structural characteristics of the welfare state only, and thus to disaggregate the activity social care from the social setting and downplay the key role of gender and power relations in a society. Daly (2002) claims to combine the two strands of research: 'care as a social good' with its embeddedness in gender and social relations prevalent in feminist research and 'care as a public good' with its focus on welfare state regulations on social care. In her research, she discusses the interrelationship between welfare state regulations and societal consequences in respect to the issue of gender equity, the appropriate welfare mix in society, the extent to which care is legitimised, the demand for and supply of labour, the appropriate welfare mix in society and the balancing of the public finances. Bettio and Plantenga (2004) also combine both strands of research and discuss the consequences of different regulations on the employment status and opportunities of women, poverty and fertility rates. Knijn and Kremer (1997) related rights and needs of care givers and care receivers shaped by welfare state regulations to the issue of gender inequality in citizenship rights.

According to Daly (2002), the debate on care as a public good clarifies issues around social care which are central to the framing and definition of home care governance. The research emphasises care delivery, existing governance arrangements (and policies) and the necessary institutional regulations as well as the situation of the users and the idea of care as a social right. The rules of access and the types of support granted are strongly related to values about the role of the families – respectively, men and women – but also regarding the fair distribution of resources. Despite a rich description of case study questions such as how the different governance arrangements are developed and implemented, on a conceptual level it is a neglected area.

Comparative Studies and Welfare State Change

Cross-country studies use social policy approaches and their societal implications to compare social care settlements and their development in different countries. Inspired by Esping-Andersen's (1990) ideas on welfare state regimes, the social care model approach organises countries into different groups on the basis of certain characteristics of their social care provision. Anttonen and Sipilä (1996) developed the first social care model on the basis of the dimensions 'way of organising' and 'volume of social care services'. They distinguish the Scandinavian model with its universal public social care services, the UK approach with (public) social services accessible after means testing, the family care model in Southern Europe with its emphasis on unpaid family care, and the Continental European subsidiary model where the family takes on primary responsibility first, but actors of the civil society replace the family if necessary.

Later, Sipilä and Anttonen (1999) related the different modes of producing social care to the consequences for care givers and care receivers in regard to the issue of social and gender inequality. As a starting-point they choose the relationship between carers and care receivers, which increases in complexity when it becomes formal as a result of the increasing number of actors. The modes of producing care, including voluntary, commercial, grey market, public or by the families, differ in regard to the financier, the mode of financing, the producing unit and the resulting consequences for carers and care receivers. In their findings they describe the typical users of different types, showing that the modes of producing care are strongly linked to class position, citizenship status or family status. Furthermore, the working situation of the carers differs according to the cash payment received or to the working conditions. Comparable to Sipilä and Anttonen, Stark and Regner (2002) examine different modes of care provision and their consequences for the carers and care receivers on the basis of three case studies (Spain, Sweden and Germany) which represent three different welfare state models. In order to reveal the consequences of the different approaches they include assessment procedures and access criteria to societal support, as well as the preferences and desires of the elderly according to the provision and the funding of care services.

By distinguishing among the types of societal support such as time, money and service, Bettio and Plantenga (2004) organised European social care approaches to different clusters. They construct an 'all in the family cluster', mainly in Southern Europe, in which care activities and the management of care are delegated to the family and the societal support on all three types is low. In the 'public financing private care cluster' in Continental Europe, a largely informal family-based care strategy is predominant which is supported by financial provision such as cash benefits and different types of leave arrangements. In the 'public care cluster', a care strategy is implemented where families are supported by a wide range of universally available services but also by generously funded leave facilities.

The development of different social care models or clusters reveals the complexity of social care governance and the variety of dimensions for an analysis to be considered. The dimensions have been extended since the beginning of the 1990s. While initially they examined funding, care sectors and their interplay and consequences for care users and carers, they gradually included more components to analyse access to the services as well as further types of support for carers and care receivers. These developments also reflect a change in social care delivery characterised by an involvement and acknowledgement of more actors in formal and informal care.

The change of welfare state regulations around care and its consequences for women's lives are at the centre of the approach of Daly and Lewis (1998). In contrast to the social care models which are concentrated on the macro level, the three dimensions they use for the analysis of social care – care as labour, care as a normative framework and care as cost – are located at the macro and micro levels. This enables one to assess restructurings on the macro level that were carried out in many Western countries during the 1990s, and their consequences for the micro-level daily care work. In their approach they use case studies to show the development and reject the idea of organising countries into different models or clusters. They argue that the development of countries traditionally assigned to one model differ substantially during the 1990s.

Daly and Lewis (1998) develop two dimensions meaningful for the analysis of change: first, they emphasise the increasing care provision within the market and the introduction of market principles in the public sector as a pathway of change towards marketisation; and second, they describe the establishment of diversified types of support, services and benefits as combined into comprehensive care arrangements in different countries as a second trend to welfare state change. They argue that the new types of regulations are established at a middle tier between the most generous levels and regulations on the social assistance level, typically means tested.

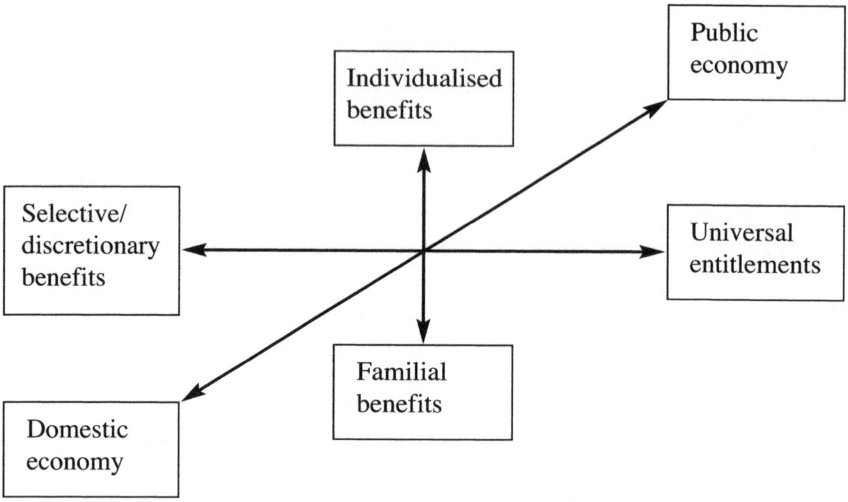

Source: Adapted from Anttonen et al. (2003: 173).

Figure 2.1 Dimensions of change in social care

The analysis of change is also at the centre of the approach of Anttonen et al. (2003) (see Figure 2.1). They define three dimensions on which they locate processes of change. In the first, 'social care going public', they describe the increasing share of care activities that have left the domestic economy of the household and are now provided as formal services in the public economy. The second and third dimensions describe regulations of access to services or benefits. Individualisation is the development from the family to the individual as allocation unit and universalisation is the development from discretionary to universal entitlements. On the basis of case studies they compared the development in the dimensions in different countries and found varying patterns of development: first, the social care delivery in general does not develop in the same direction on all three dimensions in one country; second, a different development can be observed in regard to individual benefits and services; and third, the development may differ on national and local levels.

In conclusion, cross-country studies typically examine social care governance on a macro level using characteristics of welfare state delivery such as funding, accessibility and the services covered. Only in the approach of Daly and Lewis (1998) are the macro and micro levels conceptually interwoven, thus enabling the inclusion of the relationship to daily care work. The dimensions used in this research are comparable to the dimensions described in the previous sections. When care models are created, the chosen dimensions are on a very abstract level. However, these dimensions illustrate which ones might be relevant in comparative research on home care governance and change. Although the comparisons are oriented towards care governance, the selected dimensions may be used as a starting-point for the analysis of policy developments.

THE PUBLIC POLICY LITERATURE AND THE ANALYSIS OF HOME CARE GOVERNANCE

Based on the review above, the following discussion suggests that the public policy literature can usefully complement the social care literature and contribute to a better understanding of home care governance across different countries. More specifically, the chapter argues that the public policy literature adds two important sets of explanations to the comparative analysis of home care governance: first, the literature highlights the formal institutions related to the political system and policy subsystems and as such adds a further factor shaping home care governance; and second, the literature emphasises the specific *dynamics* of home care governance and thereby offers deeper insights into the interplay between institutions and ideas.

However, using ideas taken from the public policy literature in a cross-country analysis of home care governance is not straightforward. Large parts of the public policy literature are gender blind (see Waylen, 1998) whereas, as the review of the social care literature illustrated, home care is a highly gendered area of governance. This does not mean that concepts such as actors, institutions and ideas cannot be used when analysing home care governance, but such concepts need to be gendered. The following review includes insights from feminist policy analyses, feminist studies of the state and feminist scholarship on the welfare state. This body of literature asks questions about what determines public policies concerning women, the effects of public policies on women, the relationship between feminist movements and the state, and the political representation and participation of women (for an overview, see Dahlerup, 1987). Further, reflecting the specifics of the literature, the following review focuses on the dynamics between institutions and ideas as leading to governance as both policy output and broader governing arrangements. By way of setting the scene for the following review, we first discuss the specific features of home care as a policy subsystem.

The Specifics of Home Care as a Policy Subsystem

The specific features of home care as an area of governance are closely related to its highly gendered nature. The feminist emphasis on the gender specificity of home care governance resonates with the notion of policy subsystems developed in the public policy literature (for an overview, see Jordan and Maloney, 1997). Policy subsystems suggest that policy making organises itself around specific issues or problems because the complexity and specificity of such policy issues requires some degree of division of labour. This also means that the nature of policy issues partly structures politics (as in how policies are made) or as Freeman (1985) puts it, 'policies determine politics'. A policy subsystem is the space where actors discuss a specific policy issue and bargain in pursuit of their interests. Significantly these interactions also occur in the context of sector-specific institutions and underlying ideas (see ibid.; Peters, 1992; Parsons, 1995; Howlett and Ramesh, 2003).

So, what are the specifics of home care as a policy issue and what does this mean for the characteristics of the policy subsystem of home care? The review of the social care literature in the first part of this chapter suggests that home care as a policy issue is specific in the three closely related respects: the centrality of gender, the interface between the public and the private, and the close relationship between the macro and the micro levels. This means that home care policies have different meanings and implications for women and men, are characterised by a close co-existence between the private and public spheres of work, and that different levels are tightly related.

The specific nature of home care means that as a policy issue, home care does not fit easily into the public nature of policies precisely because home care stretches the meaning of what public means (Randall, 1998; Waylen, 1998). The fact that home care tends to be associated with the private sphere means that (public) policies of home care are often limited in scope and that women and women's interests in home care are often excluded (Dahlerup, 1987). Yet public policies and the state do impact on home care and women (as carers and cared for) do influence public policies relating to home care. This illustrates the twofold position of the state: the state represents and reproduces gender relations in home care as the more or less tacitly enforced saliency of informal home care demonstrates, while the state is also the key site for renegotiating such relations. Examples of the second aspect are major reform initiatives introducing long-term care insurance in Japan and Germany since the mid-1990s which reflect cultural changes in women's lives, including the greater articulation and recognition of the claim of economic independence through participation in the labour market (see Conway et al., 1998; Briskin, 1999; Charles, 2000).

In terms of the policy subsystem of home care, this has several implications.

First, considering that existing institutional contexts have traditionally constrained rather than promoted interests in home care, the relative openness of such institutions to new ideas and actors is an important component of the policy subsystem of home care (see Lovenduski and Randall, 1993). Importantly, institutions also operate at different levels since responsibility of home care policies is often delegated to local levels (see Alber, 1995; Burau and Kröger, 2004 in relation to the UK and Finland). Second, ideas underpinning home care policies are related to both salient and new ideas about gender arrangements and as such gender makes up the basic fabric of the policy subsystem of home care. Finally, interests in home care tend to operate from the outside, reflecting the fact that while women are now in the public realm of paid work this is not matched by the development of public services (Hernes, 1987b; Briskin, 1999). This makes for a diverse range of actors, including actors operating on the outside, such as patient advocacy groups and professional carers' associations, and actors operating on the inside as advocates of patients and carers, such as provider organisations and government ministries.

The specifics of the policy subsystem of home care also requires us to consider different types of policies (Dahlerup, 1987; Waylen, 1998): policies specifically directed at women, such as those concerned with providing respite care to informal carers; policies dealing with relations between men and women, such as those defining the relative weight given to informal care; and more general policies also affecting women, such as policies emphasising the primacy of care in non-institutional settings. A final category of policies is so-called 'policy silences' (Conway et al., 1998) or implicit policies (Randall, 2000). This type resonates with Lukes's (2005) notion of non-decisions and describes the implicit or explicit decision not to take a decision. Here, the traditionally low profile of home care as a policy issue is a classic example.

Institutions and Ideas

In a now classic definition, Heidenheimer et al. describe the comparative study of public policy as the analysis of 'how, why and to what effect different governments pursue particular causes of action and inaction' (1983: 2). This suggests that, like the social care literature, the comparative study of public policy is concerned with analysing the tools of public policies (the *how* of policies) as well as the consequences of different policies (the *to what effect* of policies). Significantly, however, the public policy literature goes beyond that and also asks about the reasons for why policies look the way they do (the *why* of policies). This signals a more explicit concern with *explaining* policies in addition to mapping out policies and their effects. Not surprisingly, there is a wide range of different theories as to how public policies can be explained.

These theories can be distinguished as to the relative emphasis they put on institutions, ideas and actors. The following discussion focuses on the first two sets of theories as these are most relevant for our analysis.

One set of theories focuses on institutions as the structures in which policies are made. Theories range from *statist* approaches emphasising the structures of the state (see Skocpol, 1985) to *new institutionalist* approaches (see Hall and Taylor, 1996; Peters, 1999). Concerning the influence of the state on public policies, structures relating to *state autonomy* (the relative independence of the state from social pressures) and *state capacity* (the ability of the state to make and implement policies) are key (Howlett and Ramesh, 2003). They include the relative (de)centralisation of political power and the relative location of central power in the legislature and the executive, respectively. In contrast, institutionalist approaches look at structures more broadly and analyse institutions as formal and informal procedures and examine both organisations and the rules promulgated by organisations. Institutions are the relatively stable structures from which policies emerge, and as such often point to the most visible differences among countries. Institutions thus provide an important springboard for cross-country analyses of home care governance and for explaining differences and similarities across countries.

The feminist literature on public policy also emphasises the importance of the structures in which policies are made. Here the literature often focuses on the state and specifically on how the state both reflects existing gender relations and actively shapes such gender relations as well as women's activities (Randall, 1998; Waylen, 1998; Charles, 2000). This demonstrates the close relationship women tend to have with the state. As Hernes (1987b) points out, women are closely integrated into the spheres of private and public reproduction but do not have the same organisational buffer as men defending their interests. The state rather than the market, therefore, is central for women and for defining their position. However, feminist writings on the state have had a tendency to treat the state as a monolithic actor which is problematic considering variations across not only countries but also policy sectors (Dahlerup, 1987; Waylen, 1998). Against this background, more recent feminist literature tries to disaggregate the state and instead looks at the specific institutions related to the state and examines their enabling and constraining effects in relation to women's interests. This includes analysing conflicting interests within the state and at different levels. Waylen (1998), for example, suggests analysing the state as a gendered highly bureaucratic organisation. Similarly, Charles (2000) argues for treating the state as a state of social relations that are themselves contested. This means acknowledging the state as a highly complex entity that is both the terrain and the object of political struggles. This directs attention to the internal organisation of the state and possible variations among its different parts, as well as its changeable nature. In a similar vein, Randall (2000) introduces the notion of 'gendered institutionalism' which involves asking questions about the specific politics and policy processes in both historical and comparative perspectives. In contrast, Briskin (1999) highlights the importance of different welfare-state regimes, suggesting that they reflect differences in the political forces shaping countries and differences in more general state–society/public–private relations. Importantly, the gendered statism and institutionalism in feminist writings also points to a broader underlying understanding of institutions. In relation to home care this includes specific institutions (or gender orders, see Pfau-Effinger, 2004) relating to the gendered division of labour, including the labour market, the welfare state and the family.

What are the implications for the comparative analysis of home care governance? As relatively stable structures, institutions point to salient differences among countries and are crucial to explaining home care policies comparatively, not least as institutions enable us to analyse the specific conditions under which home care policies emerge. However, in terms of the range of institutions considered it is important to go beyond mainstream comparisons in public policy, with their focus on the state and the political system as such, and instead also analyse the specific organisational settings and procedures of home care polices as embedded in broader gender orders.

Another way of explaining public policies and variations across countries is to look at ideas understood as traditions, beliefs and attitudes about the world and society (for an overview, see Busch and Braun, 1999; Nahrath, 1999). Views about causal relations and norms form the backbone of institutions and as such also constrain the nature of policy options. At the same time, ideas also serve actors as focal points, ideational prisms or frames that help actors select among different courses of action (see Braun, 1999; Bleich, 2002). As Hall (1993) points out, ideas often constitute a policy paradigm defined as taken for granted assumptions about policy goals, related problems and how to solve them. However, ideas can also change, as powerfully demonstrated by Baumgartner and Jones's (1991) notion of 'punctuated equilibrium'.

The notion that ideas as traditions, beliefs and attitudes play an important role in shaping public policies is also implicit in the feminist literature. However, while the public policy literature focuses on the specific mechanisms by which this occurs, the feminist writings on public policy are more concerned with the substance of the ideas themselves. As the review of the social care literature above discusses, ideas centre around gender. Pfau-Effinger (2004), for example, introduces the notion of 'gender culture' which refers to deeply embedded beliefs and ideas about relations between the generations in the family and the obligations associated with these relations. As Charles (2000) points out, such gender cultures are closely related to the dominant political discourse about women and women and the home and as such mark the territory as to what is possible or considered necessary in policy terms.

In relation to the comparative study of home care governance, ideas are important in two respects: first, considering its highly gendered nature, home care policies cannot be thought of without ideas, notably ideas relating to the appropriate role of women in the care of older people in their own homes; and second, as a policy area, home care is characterised by both considerable policy continuity and policy change and ideas and their role in the making of policies allow this to be addressed.

DISCUSSION

This chapter began by introducing the notion of governance as a way to capture the complex forms of coordination typical of home care. The chapter then critically reviewed the social care and public policy literatures and discussed the respective literature's contribution to analysing home care governance. Figure 2.2 summarises the framework of the analysis.

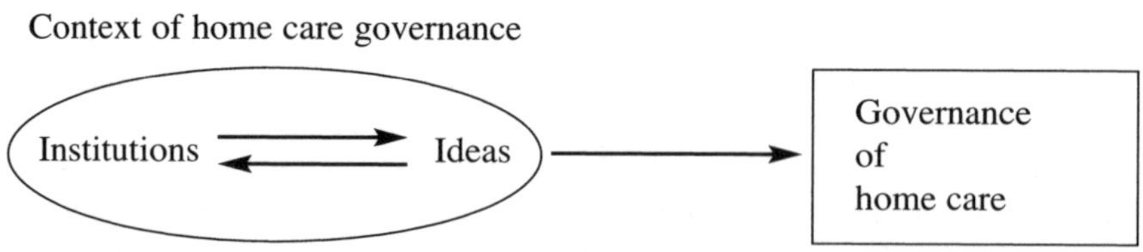

Figure 2.2 Framework for analysing the governance of home care

The review suggests that within a common focus on governance, on institutions and ideas, the two bodies of literature put different yet complementary emphases. First, they are both interested in governance arrangements as the different mechanisms (and mixes thereof) for coordinating home care. Here the social care approach is specifically concerned with coordination as related to funding and delivery, whereas the public policy approach tends to treat governance as policy output and pays greater attention to governance as rules. Second, the two literatures also share an interest in institutions and how institutions shape governance arrangements. In this respect, social care approaches are most concerned with social institution related to the family, while public policy approaches focus on formal institutions, especially the political system and institutions related to policy subsystems. Finally, the two literatures have a common interest in the role of ideas in shaping governance arrangements. The social care approaches point to the substantive dimensions of ideas as related to home care while the public policy approaches highlight the ways in which ideas matter.

The next chapter discusses how to conceptualise the context of home care governance and, more specifically, institutions and ideas as its key components, and provides a systematic analysis of the contexts of home care governance across our countries. Against this background, the subsequent substantive chapters present an analysis of central areas of the governance of home care: formal care services, informal care, care workers and the users of care. The analysis maps out governing arrangements across our countries and explores the different ways in which the specific contexts of home care governance shape governing arrangements. Based on selected case studies, the analyses also look in more detail at the interplay between specific types of institutions and ideas and consider the corresponding dynamics between key actors.

3. Contexts of governing home care: ideas and institutions

The analytical framework presented in the preceding chapter has two aims: first, to map out home care and its organisation using the concept of governance; and second, to account for differences and similarities across countries by analysing relevant ideas and institutions and the interplay between them. This provides the framework for contextualising governing arrangements across our countries.

In the conclusions of their comparative analysis of child and elderly care, Anttonen et al. (2003a) argue that using such contexts to construct typologies to systematically explain differences and similarities across countries is difficult and even problematic. The authors point to the complex dynamics of care arrangements and to the lack of standardisation of the use and provision of care services. This partly reflects the plasticity of care, that informal care can easily substitute for formal care. Instead, Anttonen et al. suggest analysing the dynamics of care arrangements within the context of the specific characteristics of individual country cases and even individual services.

Similarly our analytical model does not describe causal relations but instead a looser configuration of factors that shape the governance of home care. With several different factors at play, the effect of individual factors also partly depends on the interplay among them, thus further complicating the formulation of any precise predictions. With this in mind, the aim of the present chapter is to map out the ideas and institutions that form the context of the governance of home care in our respective countries. The substantive analyses in the following chapters provide a basis for ordering our countries in a theoretically meaningful way as well as identifying theoretically interesting cases. However, it is particularly in the specific context of individual countries that the analysis examines the extent to which ideas and institutions (and the interplay between them) help to explain governing arrangements in home care. Finally, where appropriate this chapter distinguishes among contexts as they apply to formal care services and to support for informal care, respectively, which represent the extreme points on the continuum of different arrangements in home care. This acknowledges the fact that in many ways, ideas and institutions are country specific and also vary between different substantive areas of governing.

IDEAS

As the discussion of the conceptual framework in Chapter 2 suggests, home care is a highly gendered area of governance. Both formal and informal care are provided mainly by women, and the definition of the border between both types of care giving is related to the mode of participation of women in private and public spheres in society. In terms of the ideas underpinning the governance of care-giving traditions, beliefs and attitudes about the mode of participation of men and women in society and the relations between them are therefore central.

The following analysis uses the concept of gender culture which Pfau-Effinger (2004, 2005) developed in the context of her comparative analysis of female employment and child-care arrangements. Based on different aspects related to the relations and responsibilities between generations and to the division of care work, she distinguishes among different family models and corresponding ideas on gender relations. The family models define societal assumptions about the role of the family compared to other societal institutions in the provision of care, and the underlying values concerning the gender division of labour. Three of the models are particularly relevant in relation to care of the elderly in the home: the housewife model of the male breadwinner family where care is the responsibility of the family and women are the primary carers; the female part-time carer model of the male breadwinner family where women combine care responsibility with part-time work and where care is the main responsibility of the family in part shared with the state, the market and the non-profit sector; and the dual breadwinner/institutional care model where both genders are integrated into paid employment on a full-time basis and where, based on formal care provision, the primary responsibility for care lies with the state, the market or the non-profit sector.

We add a fourth type, the dual breadwinner/female carer model, which in many ways is a liberal variant of the dual breadwinner model. Here the family is primarily responsible for care provision and women are expected to combine care responsibilities with full-time employment. The four models of gender culture point to distinct variations of the divide between the public and the private. Table 3.1 operationalises gender cultures in terms of predominant ideas about the relative state support of formal care services and informal care, respectively, on the one hand, and the relative state support of female labour market participation, on the other.

The predominant gender cultures underpinning the governance of home care across our countries cluster around one set of models: the female part-time carer model of the male breadwinner family and the dual breadwinner/female carer model. Both models assign the main responsibility

Table 3.1 Ideas underpinning the governance of home care

Country	What is the predominant model of gender culture? 1a. What are the predominant ideas about the relative state support for formal care services underlying government policies? 1b. What are the predominant ideas about the relative state support for informal care underlying government policies? 2. What are the predominant ideas about the relative state support for female labour market participation underlying government policies?
UK Female part-time carer model of the male breadwinner family	1a. *Little support* Family care to be partly shared with state and especially market and non-profit sector; based on ideas about low (welfare) stateness and 'welfare mix' 1b. *Little support* Informal care to be acknowledged, but only in part economically; based on idea of mixed economy of welfare within primacy of family care 2. *Little support* Women as part/full-time employees; based on ideas about liberalism and 'workfare'
Estonia Dual breadwinner/ female carer model	1a. *Very little support* Formal care provision very limited; based on idea of family responsibility for elder care 1b. *Some support* Economic support for informal care predominate, but only in the case of unavailability of family; based on idea of family responsibility 2. *Little support* Women as full-time employees; based on idea of gender equality in labour market but supported by state only in relation to family policy
Germany Female part-time carer model of the male breadwinner family	1a. *Little support* Only limited formal care provision especially by the non-profit sector; based on idea of family care and old/new subsidiarity 1b. *Medium support* Family care to be supported economically by the state; based on idea of family care and ideas about old/new subsidiarity

<table>
<tr><td></td><td colspan="2">2. Some support Middle-aged women as part-time employees or housewives; based on idea of freedom of choice for women between family work and labour market participation, and idea of family care</td></tr>
<tr><td>Italy Housewife model of the male breadwinner family (Southern Italy); Dual breadwinner/female carer model (Northern Italy)</td><td>Southern Italy
1a. Virtually no support Primacy of family care selectively to be shared with market; based on religious family values together with ideas about low stateness
1b. Little support Informal care to be selectively supported; based on ideas of social security/solidarity coupled with welfare mix
3. Virtually no support Women not in paid employment; based on religious family values together with ideas about low stateness</td><td>Northern Italy
1a. Little support Family care partly to be shared with state and non-profit sector and especially market (as reflected in employment of personal assistant carers); based on idea of low (welfare) stateness
1b. Little support Some regional and local support; based on idea of low (welfare) stateness
2. Little support Women as full-time employees; dual breadwinner as default option; based on idea of low (welfare) stateness</td></tr>
<tr><td>Japan Female part-time carer model of the male breadwinner family</td><td colspan="2">1a. High support Family care to be shared with state to a considerable extent; based on idea of universalism combined with old/new subsidiarity (as reflected in Gold Plan)
1b. Little support Little but increasing support for informal care; based on idea of primacy of support through formal care services
2. Some support Women as part/full-time employees; based on idea of increase labour market participation in ageing population</td></tr>
</table>

Table 3.1 continued

Country	What is the predominant model of gender culture? 1a. What are the predominant ideas about the relative state support for formal care services underlying government policies? 1b. What are the predominant ideas about the relative state support for informal care underlying government policies? 2. What are the predominant ideas about the relative state support for female labour market participation underlying government policies?
Netherlands Female part-time carer model of the male breadwinner family	1a. *High support* Family care to be shared with state to a considerable extent; based on ideas about universalism combined with old/new subsidiarity 1b. *Some support* Informal care to be acknowledged and supported, also economically; based on ideas of universalism coupled with new subsidiartiy 2. *Some support* Women as part-time employees; based on idea about increase of labour market participation
New Zealand Female part-time carer model of the male breadwinner family	1a. *Medium support* Family care to be partly shared with state and charitable trusts; based on idea of egalitarianism combined with old/new subsidiarity 1b. *Little support* Little, but increasing means-tested support of informal care; based on idea of primacy of formal care provision 2. *Some support* Women as part/full-time employees; based on focus to increase labour market participation and workfare
Sweden Dual breadwinner/institutional care model	1a. *High support* Primacy of formal care services; based on ideas of universalism and individualism, but increasing importance of idea of family support 1b. *Little support* Based on idea of primacy of formal care provision; little, but increasing support of informal care based on idea of public responsibility for care

	2. *High support* Women in full-time employment; based on idea of state-supported dual breadwinner model
US Dual breadwinner/female carer model	1a. *Little support* Family care partly to be shared with state and the non-profit sector and especially market; based on ideas of low (welfare) stateness and 'welfare mix'
	1b. *Little support* Some highly varied and limited support through programmes for indigents under Medicaid, but otherwise little support for informal care; based on idea of low (welfare) stateness and 'welfare mix'
	2. *Little support* Women as full-time employees; dual breadwinner as default option (as reflected in low social services and health insurance based on employment); based on idea of liberalism

Sources: Spence (1996); Coolen and Weekers (1998); Glendinning (1998); Knijn (1998, 2001); Simoni and Trifiletti (1998); Ashton (2000); Chamberlayne and King (2000); Trydegard (2000, 2003); Trifiletti et al. (2001); Baldock (2003); Campbell and Ikegami (2003); Centers for Medicare and Medicaid Services (2003a, b); Means et al. (2003); Saks et al. (2003); Bettio and Plantenga (2004); Japan Ministry of Health, Labour and Welfare (2004a); Pfau-Effinger (2004); Polverini and Lamura (2004); Polverini et al. (2004); Dahlberg (2005); Fargion (2005); Giullari and Lewis (2005); Sand (2005); Szebehely (2005); Kivisaar and Soots (2006).

for care provision to women within the family framework, despite labour market participation. The only exceptions are Italy and Sweden. In terms of the gendered ideas about the relative state support for formal care services and female employment, Italy is still close to the traditional housewife model of the male breadwinner family. This is especially true in the southern regions, pointing to the continued strength of religious family values together with a long tradition of weak stateness. In the northern part of the country, however, dual career families are more the norm and ideas of non-familial care are stronger (Trifiletti et al., 2001). These extreme geographical divisions reflect salient regional divisions between North and South, whereby a dual polity makes for a dual welfare policy (Fargion, 2005). In Sweden, by contrast, the dual breadwinner/institutional care model continues to be strong, and the predominant ideas underlying governance centre around extensive state support for both formal care services and female labour market participation.

The clustering around one set of models of gender culture, though, disguises interesting differences among countries, and here a distinction emerges between more liberal and more conservative variants of gender culture. Both variants are based on two complementary ideas: the idea of very selective state support directed at those in need and the idea of family care partly shared with the non-profit sector, especially the market. In the more liberal variant of gender cultures, most notably the US and the UK and de facto in Northern Italy, this reflects a strong tradition of low (welfare) stateness and liberalism that finds its more contemporary expression in ideas around the centrality of work for (personal) welfare, especially as it surfaces in workfare policies and ideas about the superiority of welfare mix. In Estonia, the idea of low (welfare) stateness concerns care for frail relatives at home only while the state strongly supports the provision of childcare to facilitate labour market participation of women. Moreover, in the US and Estonia this means that the lack of state support for home-based care makes for the de facto expectation that women engage in full-time employment while also taking on care responsibilities for frail relatives at home.

In the more conservative variant of gender cultures such as Germany, Japan and to some extent also the Netherlands, ideas around the primacy of the family as the basic unit of society and its responsibilities in relation to welfare provision are central. In its contemporary expression of new subsidiarity this means that the state does in part support women as carers and employees, but first and foremost to maintain the existing model of the female part-time carer.

Finally, there are interesting variations regarding the relative state support of formal care services and informal care, respectively. The two sets of support are closely related and the variations that exist remain under the same model of gender culture. In the Netherlands and Sweden, for example, the ideas about the relative state support have long been primarily centred on formal care services and have therefore been less strong in relation to informal care. Japan and Germany for their part are interesting examples of the very different ideational foci of newly introduced public funding schemes, with state support of formal care key in one and state support of informal care key in the other.

INSTITUTIONS

The gendered nature of home care as an area of governance requires us to consider a broad range of institutions, notably both social and political institutions. We use the typology of different care models or care regimes developed by Anttonen and Sipilä (1996) as a starting-point for capturing the social institutions underpinning the governance of home care, and combine this with Pfau-Effinger's (2004) notion of gender orders, which describes the existing structures of the gendered division of labour. This means analysing the prerequisites of such models in terms of the gendered structures of the family, the labour market and the welfare state. More specifically, we distinguish between the extent to which the state supports the delivery of formal care services and informal care giving on the one hand, and the labour market participation of women on the other. The latter type of support is important because many family carers are women of working age and because state support for female labour market participation often takes the form of welfare service employment (such as formal care services). It is interesting that in contrast to child care, the two types of support are often less well integrated in home care. In summary this makes for four models. In the public service model the state supports both types, with formal care services available universally and only some support for informal care. Women's participation in the labour market is high. Under the family care model, state support is low on both counts and the availability of formal care services is very limited, as is the support for informal care. The labour market participation of women is low. In the means-tested model, state support focuses on women in need, and publicly funded services and support of informal care are available only to the deserving (such as lone mothers and the long-term unemployed). Labour market participation of women is relatively high but not explicitly supported by the state. Under the subsidiarity model, state support for formal care services is secondary to other forms of support, especially of informal care, and state support for women's labour market participation is limited. Publicly funded services are limited and meant to support family care, and the labour market participation of women mainly takes the form of part-time employment.

In terms of the political institutions underpinning the governance of home care, the analysis focuses on the policy subsystem and especially the institutions related to the political power over both formal care services and the support of informal care. The review of feminist writing on public policy in Chapter 2 pointed to the importance of the interplay between women's agency and the state. The women's movement is generally an important indication of women's agency although specific interest in mobilisation around home care has been rare. Here old-age interest groups are in principle more relevant although these are confronted with the paradox of large numbers, but small influence. Moreover, old age often does not provide a sound basis for political mobilisation (Walker, 1999). As Campbell and Morgan (2005) in their analysis of Germany and the US suggest, the chronically ill and their carers are unlikely to be engines for policy change. Although pursuing different interests, proxy actors and especially the state offer important sources for potential alliance and political exchange (Schulte, 1999; Bonoli, 2005). At the same time the resources of the state vary, depending on the specific characteristics of the policy subsystem. In this respect Alber (1995), in his analysis of formal care services, suggests that especially the relative (vertical) (de)centralisation together with the (horizontal) cohesive-ness of political power are key.

The governance of home care has traditionally been local but is now firmly positioned in the context of central–local relations. This makes for tensions over issues of control and funding where central and local levels have different interests and resources. For example, as demonstrated by Campbell and Morgan's (2005) analysis of long-term care politics in Germany and the US, the tensions between local and national levels of government can provide an important lever for policy change. In relation to the expansion of formal care services more generally, Anttonen et al. suggest that '[s]ocial care provision rarely progresses to the status of citizenship entitlements without becoming a centralized, national government responsibility' (2003b: 191). Table 3.2 provides an overview of the social and political institutions relating to the governance of formal care service.

The discussion of the ideas underpinning the governance of home care has already hinted at the close connection between gender cultures and care regimes as the corresponding social institutions. The idea of the housewife model tends to express itself in a family care regime, the liberal and the conservative variants of the part-time female carer model of the male breadwinner family and the dual breadwinner/female carer model in a means-tested and a family care regime, respectively, and the idea of the dual breadwinner/institutional care model in a public service regime.

At the same time there are interesting hybrids. In the Netherlands, for example, the social institutions relating to formal care services follow the model of the public service care regime. State support is extensive, resulting in high-level and universally available services. This contrasts with those

Table 3.2 Institutions relating to the governance of formal care services

Country	Care regime predominant regime: Public service model, family care model, means-tested model, subsidiarity model? (in terms of the relative state support 1. for formal care services and 2. for female labour market participation)	Type of policy subsystem Political power over formal care services: Extent of (de)centralisation and cohesiveness? (in terms of 1. regulation and 2. funding)
UK	Means-tested model 1. Formal care services: social care services are means tested, scope of health care services is limited; result: considerable reliance on family care complemented by privately paid services 2. Female labour market participation: state support only for 'problem groups' (such as lone mothers, long-term unemployed); result: middle-range labour market participation with considerable part-time employment	Centralised and cohesive 1. Regulation: central government decides on overall framework (such as for quality and performance standards); specification through central regulatory bodies 2. Funding: central government allocates funds to local authorities (social care) and care trusts (health care); some local autonomy concerning allocation of funding
Estonia	Family care model 1. Formal care services: availability of social and health care services limited, especially in the rural areas; result: heavy reliance on family care 2. Female labour market participation: state support limited; result: high female labour market participation and low level of part-time work	Strongly decentralised and cohesive 1. Regulation: national government decides on framework regulating social care services and also more specific regulation for health care services; local authorities responsible for more specific regulation of social care services (e.g., eligibility, costs)

Table 3.2 continued

Country	Care regime predominant regime: Public service model, family care model, means-tested model, subsidiarity model? (in terms of the relative state support 1. for formal care services and 2. for female labour market participation)	Type of policy subsystem Political power over formal care services: Extent of (de)centralisation and cohesiveness? (in terms of 1. regulation and 2. funding)
		2. National government decides on funding for health care services, local authorities decide on funding for social care services
Germany	Subsidiarity model 1. Formal care services: social care services available as supplement, health care universally available on basis of need but limited in scope; result: predominance of family care 2. Female labour market participation: only limited state support of care services; result: middle-range female labour market participation with high part-time employment	Decentralised and cohesive 1. Regulation: federal government decides on long-term care insurance law (basic definitions on need and types and amount of benefits); statutory self-administration of insurance funds and providers decide on more specific regulation 2. Funding: within federal framework organisations of insurance funds and providers decide on funding through state-level contracts
Italy	Family care model 1. Formal care services: social care services are means tested and often not available, scope of public health services universal but limited by long waiting lists and low quality (especially in the South); result: extremely sparse public	Highly decentralised and fragmented 1. Regulation: local authorities decide on organisation of social care services; regional government decides on organisation of health care services 2. Funding: taxes formally collected by national

	services and instead predominance of privately paid individual carers 2. Female labour market participation: state support virtually non-existent, but regional support is available in some northern regions; result: low rate of labour market participation and mostly full time in the south, and much higher female activity rate in the North, increasingly also part time	government and some influence through National Fund; regional government decides on allocation and funding for health care services, and on funding of social care services; local government decides on allocation of funding of social care services
Japan	Subsidiarity model 1. Formal care services: health and social care services are available universally, co-payment but waived for low income; result: high level of services, but thorough certification process to qualify for access to services 2. Female labour market participation: state support is moderate, focused on increasing general employment rate to offset ageing population; result: especially young women likely to be in full-time employment	Decentralised and cohesive 1. Regulation: local authorities decide on organisation of social care services; regional government decide on organisation of health care services but under national guidelines 2. Funding: local authorities decide on funding of social care services, regional government decides on funding of health care services
Netherlands	Public service model 1. Formal care services: health and social care services are available universally; but increasingly support of family care required; result: high level of services, but under challenge	Centralised and cohesive 1. Regulation: central government sets criteria for micro-level allocation and quality standards 2. Funding: central government sets budgetary framework, Health Care Insurance Board allocates budgets and controls funding

Table 3.2 continued

Country	Care regime predominant regime: Public service model, family care model, means-tested model, subsidiarity model? (in terms of the relative state support 1. for formal care services and 2. for female labour market participation)	Type of policy subsystem Political power over formal care services: Extent of (de)centralisation and cohesiveness? (in terms of 1. regulation and 2. funding)
Netherlands	Subsidiarity model 2. Female labour market participation: state support limited and recent, focused on increasing general employment rate; result: middle range labour market participation with very high part-time employment	
New Zealand	Means-tested model 1. Formal care services: some social care services are means tested and others are universal, scope of health care services is broad; result: considerable reliance on family care complemented by privately paid and charitable services 2. Female labour market participation: extensive state support but largely for targeted groups such as single mothers and long-term unemployed; result: middle-range labour market participation with considerable part/full-time employment	Centralised and cohesive 1. Regulation: central government decides on overall framework (such as for quality and performance standards); specification through central regulatory bodies 2. Funding: central government allocates funds to local authorities (social care) and health authorities; some local autonomy but centralised system of accountability

Sweden	Public service model 1. Formal care services: social care services mainly available universally, but increasingly means tested, health care services available universally on the basis of need; result: formal care services but also some reliance on family support 2. Female labour market participation: high state support, result: high female labour market participation with high level of part-time employment	Strongly decentralised and cohesive 1. Regulation: national government sets basic norms of societal responsibility on home nursing and social care; local authorities decide on local goals and rules for implementation 2. Funding: local authorities decide on funding
US	Means-tested model 1. Formal care services: social care services are generally means tested, scope of health care services is limited; result: considerable reliance on family care complemented by privately paid services or private long-term care insurance 2. Female labour market participation: little state support except for targeted groups such as single mothers, school dropouts and long-term unemployed; result: high labour market participation with considerable full-time employment	Highly decentralised and fragmented 1. Regulation: local/state authorities decide on organisation of social care services; federal, state and local governments share decisions on organisation of health care services for elderly with heavy influence of private insurers and medical professions 2. Funding: local/state authorities decide on the funding of social care services; state and federal authorities decide on funding of health services

Sources: Spence (1996); Coolen and Weekers (1998); Glendinning (1998); Knijn (1998, 2001); Trifiletti (1998); Alber and Schölkopf (1999); Ashton (2000); Chamberlayne and King (2000); New Zealand Ministry of Health (2000, 2002a, 2003); Trydegard (2000, 2003); Eto (2001); European Observatory on Health Care Systems (2001); Japan Ministry of Health, Labour and Welfare (2002, 2004b); SOS (2002); Baldock (2003); Campbell and Ikegami (2003); Centers for Medicare and Medicaid Services (2003a, b); Means et al. (2003); Saks et al. (2003); European Observatory on Health Systems and Policies (2004); Polverini et al. (2004); Theobald (2004); Rauch (2005); Ministero del Lavoro e delle Politiche Sociali (2005); Kivisaar and Soots (2006).

institutions relating to female labour participation that follow the model of the subsidiarity care regime. State support for women in the labour market is limited, and this results in middle-range labour market participation with a very high share of part-time employment. This hybrid form also points to the fact that social institutions are subject to change. The introduction of the insurance for exceptional medical risks (which includes home care services) in the late 1960s marked the introduction of universalist elements into an otherwise conservative welfare state (Knijn, 2001). As such, the insurance compensated for the weakening of the traditional divisions in Dutch society (de-pillarisation) (Alber, 1995). Similarly, with the introduction of social insurance schemes for long-term care in Japan and Germany in the 1990s, the relative state support for formal care services has increased. Yet especially in Germany, relative state support continues to be hemmed in by a conservative gender culture, and formal care services are first and foremost meant to support and thereby maintain family care.

In terms of the institutions related to the policy subsystem of home care across our countries, the political power over formal care services relative to both regulation and funding is characterised by a considerable degree of decentralisation, not least reflecting the strength of the historical legacy of local governance. This resonates with Anttonen et al.'s (2003b: 192) observation that because of the tight historical links with local poor law, social care has often not been subject to decisions in the arena of democratic politics. Instead, social care has the character of a service whose development is decided by professionals and managers involved in service delivery. The subcentral level to which power is decentralised varies, however. Power rests at the local level in Sweden and Estonia, at the regional level in Germany, and at both local and regional levels in Italy and Japan, whereas in the US the distribution of power is even more complex. This evidence points to the importance of relative degree of cohesiveness as another important characteristic of political power over formal care services. Here as well as in Italy (but in contrast to the other countries mentioned above) different subcentral levels (together with the central level) exist side by side but are not integrated. By contrast, political power is more centralised in the UK, New Zealand and the Netherlands. In relation to the first two, this resonates with a highly centralised political–administrative system, whereas in the Netherlands a unitary and hierarchically flanked social insurance system makes for centralised political power.

As in the case of the ideas, the social and political institutions underpinning the governance of the support of informal care are broadly similar to those of the governance of formal care services. Nevertheless there are interesting differences that relate to the specific organisation of the relative state support of informal care giving. Table 3.3 gives an overview.

Table 3.3 Institutions relating to the governance of support of informal care

Country	Regime of care Predominant regime: public service model, family care model, means-tested model, subsidiarity model? (in terms of the relative state support 1. for informal care and 2. for female labour market participation (see Table 3.2)	Type of policy subsystem Political power over support of informal care: extent of (de)centralisation and cohesiveness? (in terms of 1. regulation and 2. funding)
UK	Means-tested model 1. Support of informal care mainly means tested but through variety of forms 2. Female labour market participation	Multi-level and fragmented Invalid Carers Allowance: funded centrally through national insurance contributions and regulated centrally by government ministry and its agencies; care vouchers/direct payments: funded centrally through grants allocated from central government to local authorities, regulated centrally through general guidelines by government ministry; complemented by more specific regulation at local level
Estonia	Family care model 1. Economic support for family care on basis of primacy of family responsibility and only in case of non-availability of family care 2. Female labour market participation	Multi-level and fragmented 1. Regulation: economic benefits decided at national and local levels 2. Funding: economic benefits funded at local level
Germany	Subsidiarity model 1. Economic support of informal care as predominant support strategy based on the ideas of family care and subsidiarity 2. Female labour market participation	Multi-level and fragmented 1. Regulation: federal government decides on basic definitions of need, types and amount of benefits 2. Funding: economic benefits funded by social insurance (federal level)

Table 3.3 continued

Country	Regime of care Predominant regime: public service model, family care model, means-tested model, subsidiarity model? (in terms of the relative state support 1. for informal care and 2. for female labour market participation (see Table 3.2)	Type of policy subsystem Political power over support of informal care: extent of (de)centralisation and cohesiveness? (in terms of 1. regulation and 2. funding)
Italy	Family care model 1. Little support of informal care, predominantly through economic benefits (at national, but increasingly also at regional and local levels) 2. Female labour market participation	Highly decentralised and fragmented with pocket of centralisation Invalid Carers Allowance: funded and regulated centrally
Japan	Subsidiarity model with means testing for cash benefits 1. Support of informal care through care services: health and social care services are available universally with 10% co-payment; in those few local authorities that provide cash payments they are means tested 2. Female labour market participation	Decentralised and cohesive 1. Regulation: local authorities decide on organisation of social care services; regional government decide on organisation of health care services but under national guidelines 2. Funding: local authorities decide on funding of social care services; a few local authorities give limited means-tested cash payments
Netherlands	Public service model 1. Support of informal care predominantly through publicly funded services and to a lesser extent economic benefits Subsidiarity model 2. Female labour market participation	Centralised and cohesive Care budget: funded and regulated centrally through social insurance for exceptional medical risks

New Zealand	Means-tested/subsidiarity model 1. Support of informal care mainly through care services: some care services are universal and others are means-tested, scope of health care services is broad; ongoing review of local inconsistencies. 2. Female labour market participation	Centralised and cohesive 1. Regulation: central government decides on overall framework (such as for quality and performance standards); specification through central regulatory bodies 2. Funding: central government allocates funds to local authorities; some local autonomy but centralised system of accountability
Sweden	Public service model 1. Predominance of support through public services; economic benefits restricted 2. Female labour market participation	Strongly decentralised and cohesive 1. Regulation: municipalities decide whether to provide economic support and if so, what criteria to use 2. Funding: municipalities decide on funding
US	Means-tested model 1. Support of informal care through care services: social care services are means tested, scope of health care services is limited; considerable reliance on family care complemented by privately paid services or private long-term care insurance 2. Female labour market participation	Highly decentralised and fragmented 1. Regulation: local/state authorities decide on organisation of social care services; federal, state and local governments share decisions on organisation of health care services for elderly with heavy influence of private insurers and medical professions 2. Funding: no cash payments by government but some long-term private plans include limited cash payments

Sources: Spence (1996); Coolen and Weekers (1998); Glendinning (1998); Knijn (1998, 2001); Trifiletti (1998); Alber and Schölkopf (1999); Ashton (2000); Chamberlayne and King (2000); New Zealand Ministry of Health (2000, 2002a); Trydegard (2000, 2003); Eto (2001); European Observatory on Health Care Systems (2001); SOS (2002); Baldock (2003); Campbell and Ikegami (2003); Centers for Medicare and Medicaid Services (2003a, b); Means et al. (2003); Saks et al. (2003); Bettio and Plantenga (2004); European Observatory on Health Systems and Policies (2004); Feltenius (2004); Japan Ministry of Health, Labour and Welfare (2004b); Polverini et al. (2004); Theobald (2004); Rauch (2005); Kivisaar and Soots (2006).

In relation to political institutions, for example in the UK, the political power over the support of informal care is divided between the national and the local levels of government. The former sets overall policy and formulates specific guidance, while the latter decides on the specific arrangements relating to the funding and regulation of the support of informal care. This makes for political power that is multi-level and fragmented and reflects the fact that in comparison to formal care services, the support of the informal falls more or less exclusively within the realm of social care. The situation in Estonia is similar, and here the broader range of services-in-kind available means that political power includes to a greater extent the local level. Italy presents the opposite case where, as compared to formal care services, the central level has some political power over support of informal care. This reflects the fact that central government is responsible for the funding and regulation of the disability allowance as the predominant form of support of informal care.

There are also interesting differences in relation to the social institutions. In the Netherlands, the public service model formally forms the basis of the support of informal care giving, with formal care services as the predominant form of support of informal care. However, the introduction of care budgets in the early 1990s marked not only the growing importance of alternative forms of support but also the creeping institutionalisation of the principle of subsidiarity (Knijn, 2001). This corresponds to the fact that historically the public service model has evolved in close association with the delivery of formal services, initially in relation to residential settings. The further the care of older people has moved from this origin the weaker the public service model, not least also pointing to the tensions underpinning the co-existence of the principles of universality and subsidiarity. The situation in Japan and New Zealand is similar, where means-tested cash benefits and the limited public forms of support make for more strongly hybrid models of care regimes. In both cases this reflects the fact that the relative state support is predominantly directed at formal care services.

CONCLUSIONS

This chapter has specified ideas and institutions as the context of the governance of home care. So how do institutions as reflected in care regimes and policy subsystems, together with gender cultures as underlying ideas, shape the governance of home care? As suggested earlier, the governance of home care is a highly politicised and dynamic area of governance. The care regimes, together with the gender cultures, provide a basis for different (substantive) pathways of governing home care. The specific focus of such pathways varies between different areas of governance as the substantive chapters on formal care services and care workers, informal care and care users will demonstrate. The characteristics of the policy subsystem (in conjunction with the corresponding constellations of actors) also make certain pathways more likely than others, and can indicate the relative balance between continuity and change as well as the likelihood of pathbreaking change.

4. Governing formal care services: between integration and fragmentation

Within the overall context of governing home care, the area of formal care services has an ambivalent position. Compared to other areas of governance, particularly informal care, formal care services are much less inclusive in quantitative terms. As Table 4.1 illustrates, across our countries the expenditure on formal care services is well under 1 per cent of GDP and thus well below the expenditure on other welfare services such as health care. Yet

Table 4.1 Expenditure on long-term home care as a percentage of GDP, 2000

Country	Total long-term care[1] expenditure
Estonia	n/a
Germany	0.47
Italy	0.58[2]
Japan	0.02
Netherlands	0.61
New Zealand	0.12
Sweden	0.82
UK	0.41
US	0.33

Notes

1. The notion of 'long-term care' used in a national context can be substantially broader, e.g., by including residential homes for older people (e.g. Netherlands, Nordic countries).
2. Estimated public spending on long-term care (1992–95) as a percentage of GDP. Long-term care spending refers to the care needed to help older persons to lead an independent life, at home or in an institution. It excludes informal help. For home care, it should include all home care services, including district nurse services, excluding medical visits. For institutions, it includes all the costs related to care and lodging, including help for all self-care activities, but excluding medical costs.

Source: International Reform Monitor (nd); OECD (2005b).

Table 4.2 Public and private expenditure on long-term home care as a percentage of GDP, 2002

Country	Public long-term care expenditures	Private long-term care expenditures
Estonia	n/a	n/a
Germany	0.43	0.04
Italy	n/a	n/a
Japan	0.25	0.00
Netherlands	0.56	0.05
New Zealand	0.11	0.01
Sweden	0.78	0.04
UK	0.32	0.09
US	0.17	0.16

Note: The notion of 'long-term care' used in a national context can be substantially broader, e.g., by including residential homes for older people (e.g., Netherlands, Nordic countries). Public costs include all costs incurred by public institutions, municipalities, sickness funds or old-age funds. Private spending refers to out-of-pocket payments or payments by private long-term care insurance when the definitions are available.

Sources: Germany: OECD Health Data 2004; US: OECD Health Data 2004; Japan, New Zealand, UK and Sweden: Secretariat estimates based on replies to the OECD questionnaire on long-term care.

formal care services are the area of home care governance that engenders the most political debate for a number of reasons. Funding from public sources and provision by paid care workers means that formal care services are clearly visible and resemble other welfare services. As Table 4.2 demonstrates, with the exception of the US, across our countries public expenditure is by far the main source of funding for formal care services.

The ambivalent position of formal care services in relation to home care as a whole is coupled with a double division within services themselves between health and social care on the one hand and public and private provision on the other. As such, formal care services well encapsulate a central and salient tension in the governance of home care: the tension between integration and fragmentation. This chapter analyses governing arrangements in relation to formal care services in terms of the relative degrees of integration and fragmentation, looking at governing through provision, funding and rules. From a cross-country perspective, the chapter also explores which types of ideas and institutions provide more or less favourable conditions for relatively integrated governing arrangements.

GOVERNING FORMAL CARE SERVICES THROUGH DELIVERY: VARIATIONS OF THE DOUBLE FRAGMENTATION

Formal care services include a wide variety of services. Moreover, the variety of the substantive focus of services is closely related to a variety of the organisation of services, and this has a number of implications for the governance of formal care services. Formal care services in home care have to deal with both health care and social care related needs, yet in many countries the two types of needs fall into the responsibility of separately organised services. This makes for considerable fragmentation, not least as the division in terms of the delivery is often mirrored in divisions in terms of the funding of services. Another related type of fragmentation arises from the fact that different types of providers (notably public and private for- and non-profit providers) often exist side by side. In part, this is related to the first type of fragmentation, since health care services are often more likely to be in the hands of public providers, reflecting a firmer embeddedness in the welfare state. Considering this double fragmentation, issues surrounding the integration of formal care services are the focus of governing service delivery. In principle, the likelihood of integration is higher where delivery is public and lower where delivery is private.

The discussion of the context of the governance of home care in Chapter 3 suggests that variations across countries, especially concerning the relative balance between public and private provision, are related to the specific nature of ideas and institutions underpinning governing arrangements. For example, a care culture based on the idea of care as a public responsibility, such as the dual breadwinner/institutional care model, provides a favourable basis for public provision. The same applies to a care regime that gives primacy to formal care services, as is the case in the public service model. Both signal in principle an extensive public commitment to the provision of formal care services. Similarly coherent if not centralised political power over formal care services may be an important precondition for public service provision because it is closely related to the resources of the state. Governing formal care services through service delivery is associated with a diverse set of arrangements. Table 4.3 gives an overview of the variants of the double fragmentation in governing arrangements.

The UK, Estonia, Italy and New Zealand are examples of the first set of variations where the delivery of health and social care services is separate, making for a certain degree of fragmentation of governing through delivery. More specifically, public providers tend to be dominant in health care services while private non- and for-profit providers prevail in social care services, reflecting the often firmer institutionalisation of health care services in welfare

Table 4.3 Delivery of formal care services

Organisation of services	Predominant type of provider		
	Public	Private non-profit/for-profit	Mixed
Separate health care services	UK Italy New Zealand	Estonia	Japan US
Separate social care services	Estonia	UK New Zealand	Italy Japan US
Integrated health and social care services	Sweden	Germany Netherlands	

states. In the UK, the so-called 'health and social care divide' has been a salient feature of the delivery of formal care services (Means et al., 2003). Health care services are part of the National Health Service (NHS) and delivered publicly by community care trusts and more recently primary care trusts led by general practitioners. In contrast, social care local authorities are responsible for the commissioning of services, while the delivery lies in the hands of a variety of public and increasingly private providers (Forder et al., 2004). This reflects the introduction of the purchaser–provider split in the early 1990s and the associated emphasis on welfare mix, which makes for a double fragmentation of services (Land and Lewis, 1998). As a result, the availability of services is uneven (Brodhurst and Glendinning, 2001). The development fits in well with a care regime where the boundary between public and private responsibilities is blurred, as is typical of the means-tested model.

The pattern in the UK is also embedded in ideas about low or at least uncertain welfare stateness. The hollowing-out entitlements to tax-funded health care service, together with the redefinition of care needs as social care services that come with high co-payments, has heightened the fragmentation between the two services (Lewis, 2001). This also illustrates the linkage between the public/private and the health care/social care divisions. Not surprisingly, recent policy initiatives aim to foster a closer integration of formal care services. The newly created primary care trusts have more explicit mandatory responsibilities in relation to the coordination of health and social care services, and are envisaged to eventually incorporate both types of formal care services (Hudson and Henwood, 2002).

In Estonia, the delivery of social and health care is also fragmented, although it takes on a different form (see Kivisaar and Soots, 2006). The introduction of the national health insurance after independence has been combined with service delivery by private for-profit and non-profit providers. This includes family practitioner practices, self-employed nurses, hospitals run by charitable organisations and private companies. In contrast, within the area of social care administered at the local level public delivery prevails, although in some of the larger towns private non-profit providers may also exist. Considering that this arrangement of services only occurred since the 1990s, the availability of social and home nursing services is often limited, especially in rural areas (Saks et al., 2003). In short, there are not only many different types of providers but national and local levels of governing often function side by side. Taken together, this makes for a considerable level of fragmentation of service delivery.

In many ways the situation in Italy mirrors that in the UK and Estonia, although there are additional layers of geographical fragmentation (Trifiletti, 1998; Polverini et al., 2004) that point to the importance of the relative cohesion of political power over formal care services. The delivery of health care services is part of the national health service and as such, providers are predominantly public. In principle, public delivery makes for high integration. However, in the case of Italy home health care services are not only tightly limited to medically-related services but there are also considerable geographical variations, since the funding and organisation of services is in the hands of regions. Regions in the North are characterised by a much higher level of service provision than regions in the South (Polverini and Lamura, 2004). The fragmentation is even stronger in relation to social care services. Municipalities are responsible for the organisation and funding of services (although there is often little planning; see Trifiletti, 1998) while the delivery of services is entrusted to a mix of public and private non-profit providers, especially care cooperatives. Again, service delivery is patchy and limited in scope (with the exception of a few regions mainly concentrated in the North of the country).

In summary, multiple fragmentation makes for a general lack of availability of formal care services (Convery and Cioni, 2001; Simoni and Trifiletti, 2005) and reflects a number of factors. Political power over formal care services is not only highly decentralised but also lacks cohesion. Instead it is highly fragmented, with responsibilities spread across different levels and areas of services. Furthermore, especially in the South, ideas on the primacy of family care are still dominant – typically the housewife model of the male breadwinner family. The Italian welfare state has also traditionally focused on providing social support in the form of monetary transfers rather than by means of direct service delivery (Polverini and Lamura, 2004). The lack of availability of formal care services combined with changing patterns of family life and female employment has led to the emergence of a strong element of private provision, often in the form of migrant carers individually employed and paid for by families. Indeed, this has become the second most important pillar in the care mix after informal care (Polverini et al., 2004).

In terms of variations across countries, Sweden emerges as a classical example of the logic of the state, and the integration of delivery is very high. Sweden is the only one among our countries where health and social care services are integrated and where both services are in the hands of public providers. The last aspect resonates with a care regime that gives primacy to formal care service typical of the public service model. In the case of Sweden, this is further strengthened by a gender culture that combines ideas of individualism and universalism. In this model, universal access to formal care services is seen as the central means to secure the independence of individual citizens, both older people and women in paid employment. Additionally, in half of the localities county councils have delegated the responsibility for home nursing to municipalities (National Board of Health and Welfare, 2000). This makes for highly integrated service provision since municipalities also provide social care-oriented home help services. An insufficient increase of funding, however, has limited the development of service integration. Earlier hospital discharge has increased the care needs and this has taken up a much higher proportion of the care resources than anticipated. As a consequence, the municipalities have focused on service delivery for the severely care-dependent elderly and have neglected services for the elderly with only minor needs (Trydegard, 2003). In addition, opening up the care sector for private providers within the framework of an emerging ideology of welfare mix has put the existing system under pressure. The number of non-public providers delivering home care for municipalities increased by 146 per cent between 1995 and 1998 (National Board of Health and Welfare, 2000) although the overall number remains small.

The relative integration of services is less strong in Germany and the Netherlands. Although health and social care services are integrated in both countries, private non-profit providers have traditionally dominated the provision of health and social care services. This mainly reflects the strength of ideas surrounding subsidiarity in the context of a gender culture based on the female part-time care model of the male breadwinner family. Subsidiarity gives preference to care provided by civil society as opposed to public provision by the state. In both countries, the logic of associations is increasingly complemented by the logic of the market, leading to the rise of for-profit providers.

In the Netherlands, the delivery of formal care services is in the hands of non-profit organisations, regional so-called 'Cross' associations. The associations go back to earlier denominational organisations that gradually became integrated into the publicly funded and regulated delivery of services. In the past, separate organisations existed for home nursing and home help services but in the early 1990s the two started to merge with the aim of increasing the efficiency of service delivery (Kerkstra and Hutten, 1996). Similarly, only one organisation used to operate in any one area and taken together this made for a high degree of integration of service delivery. However, this began to change in the 1990s, when the government introduced market mechanisms and a mixed economy of care (Knijn, 1998). The government earmarked public funds to support private providers and required all providers to negotiate contracts with the central insurance agency. Altogether this has led to a considerable fragmentation of service delivery, reflecting the deep tensions between the different logics of governance underpinning the reforms combined.

Similar to the Netherlands, Germany has traditionally been a classical example of the dominance of non-profit providers. However, the introduction of the long-term care insurance ended the dominance of the five main non-profit providers and led to the mushrooming of alternative private providers. The number of providers of home care has increased from 4300 in 1992 to 12 700 in 2003, and 52 per cent of providers were privately owned in 2001 (Cuellar and Wiener, 2000: 18–25; Theobald, 2004). The higher levels of service provision do not necessarily make for greater diversity of services because delivery is strictly oriented towards the services covered by the long-term care and health insurance (Theobald, 2004). Despite an improved integration of nursing and personal care services, the sharp separation between ambulatory and hospital care continues to exist (Wasem, 1997; Theobald, 2004).

The types of providers involved in the delivery of formal care services are more mixed in the US and Japan. Together with separate health and social care services, this makes for a high degree of fragmentation, especially in the US. Although Medicare funding of home health services doubled between 1987 and 1996 and is expected to grow at an annual rate of at least 9 per cent (Kadushin, 2004), formal care services remain highly fragmented and are characterised by wide variations in terms of the types of providers and the degrees to which health and social care services are integrated from one locality and state to another. Not surprisingly, private long-term care insurance is big business in the US but most such policies offer only limited home care benefits (Delevett, 1999; Wenger, 2004). Similar to Italy, this points to the fact that political power over formal care services is not only highly decentralised but also highly fragmented and spread across local, state and federal levels and with different programmes existing side by side.

In contrast, in Japan political power over formal care services is more cohesive and the responsibilities at local and regional levels are embedded in a national framework and complement each other. Under the long-term insurance plan, municipalities as the insurers of the long-term care insurance have the responsibility of promoting the health and welfare of the elderly at home. Nevertheless, municipalities contract with a wide variety of organisations, including private-sector companies, for home care. This reflects a specific design feature of the insurance, notably the fact that care users access services based on an individual long-term care service usage plan and can make use of public and private medical care and welfare services comprehensively. They can choose the type of service and facilities they desire from services provided by various organisations, such as private companies, agricultural cooperatives, livelihood cooperatives, volunteer organisations and so forth.

What emerges is a picture of fragmentation of governing through delivery in the form of variations of the double fragmentation between health/social care services on the one hand and public/private providers on the other. The variations are related to contextual factors that support provision by non-public providers (as the idea of subsidiarity in the case of Germany and the Netherlands) and that means that political power lacks cohesion (adding further layers of fragmentation) as in the cases of Italy and the US.

GOVERNING FORMAL CARE SERVICES THROUGH FUNDING: VARIATIONS OF THE SETTLEDNESS OF PUBLIC FUNDING

The governance of formal care services through funding centres around arrangements relating to how formal care services are paid. The variants that exist mirror those in other welfare services and include public funding through taxes and social insurance, private funding through private donations (reflecting the logic of associations) and private insurance together with out-of-pocket payments (reflecting the logic of the market). The relative degree of (de)centralisation of responsibility for funding and the relative degree of integration of funding for health and social care services cut across the existing variants. More specifically, the variants of governing through funding make for different degrees of settledness of governing through funding, understood as more or less stable arrangements for funding formal care services that allow for more or less institutionalised access to funding.

What are the possible explanations for different degrees of settledness of governing through funding? The settledness of funding is likely to be higher in the case of public funding either through taxes or social insurance than through private funding, not least as the latter is often based on a portfolio of sources, some of which, like out-of-pocket payments, are potentially unstable.

The relative integration of funding of health and social care services is closely related to the relative integration of governing through delivery. The integration of funding arrangements potentially further strengthens the settledness of governing through funding. The effect of the relative (de)centralisation of responsibility for funding is more ambivalent and, as discussed in relation to governing through delivery, the relative horizontal concentration or cohesion of funding arrangements may be particularly important. As Table 4.4 suggests, the logic of state looms large and, with the exception of social care services in the US, in all other cases different forms of public funding exist. Therefore variations of public funding arrangements are particularly interesting.

Table 4.4 Funding of formal care services

Organisation of funding	Predominant type of funding		
	Taxes	Social insurance	Private
Separately for health care services	UK Italy (regional/ national) New Zealand	Germany US (Medicare) Japan Estonia	
Separately for social care services	UK (local) Italy (local/ regional) New Zealand Estonia	Germany Japan (local)	US
For both health and social care services	Sweden (local)	Netherlands	

In the UK, Italy, New Zealand and Sweden, formal care services are tax funded. In principle, this makes for a high degree of settledness of governing through funding because tax funding is often closely related to the idea of more or less strong universal access. However, there is considerable variation across countries, thus confirming that specific variations among different forms of public funding are particularly important here. In the case of the UK, for example, access to health and social care services is very different despite both being tax funded. Health care services are part of the NHS and free at the point of use, whereas local authorities are responsible for social care services which are means tested. Over the last decade, more and more services have been defined as social rather than health care and as such incur charges. Combined with targeting of services by local authorities, this also means that older people increasingly have to rely on either their own funds or the help of family and friends in order to pay for services and stay in their own homes (Baldock, 2003). Glendinning (1998; similarly Brodhurst and Glendinning, 2001) suggests that this strategy has led to considerable reduction of citizenship rights in what until the 1980s was a universal system. As noted above, recent developments also resonate with a care regime where the boundary between public and private responsibilities is blurred, which is typical of the means-tested model. The case of the UK is also embedded in ideas about low (or at least uncertain) welfare stateness.

Like the UK, in Sweden the targeting of social services has also enlarged and is increasingly oriented towards highly care-dependent elderly with limited family support. Considering the very different context of the governance of home care in Sweden, this is a significant change and marks a retreat from the ideas of universalism and individualism that are characteristic of the Swedish gender culture. Reforms in the 1990s aimed at strengthening social care and at integrating social and nursing/health care, crucially under the premise of a social model. However, the limited increase of funds at the local level, combined with a policy of early hospital discharge, in effect shifted the balance between the delivery of nursing and social care in favour of the former (Trydegard, 2003).

By comparison, developments in New Zealand seem to be going in the opposite direction. Since the early 1990s, public policy has supported a philosophy of 'ageing in place', and strategies have included increasing public expenditure on home care and support services. Home support expenditure more than doubled between 1995/96 and 2002/03 from NZ$60 million to NZ$148 million (New Zealand Ministry of Health, 2003a: 40). The government partially or fully subsidises a wide range of home care services, particularly those that depend upon professional expertise, such as nursing. Eligibility and level of service are determined by needs assessment. These recent developments are typical of a care regime that combines very limited universality with means testing and where privately paid and charitable services complement family care. In relation to the last aspect, it is also indicative that there are some additional community support services that are not publicly funded, such as transportation, which are also often provided free of charge to persons in need. The main source of funds for these services is the Lottery Grants Board, which provides funds to not-for-profit organisations.

With social insurance funding in Germany, Japan and the Netherlands, home care is an individually earned right although individual benefits are often needs based. The public funding of home care has traditionally been less well established in social insurance systems. This resonates with a gender culture that has traditionally been very strongly based on the ideal of family care and women as housewives or part-time employees. Both Germany and

Japan, however, have seen the introduction of separate social insurance schemes dedicated to long-term care and as such the settledness of governing through funding has increased considerably.

Under Japan's New Ten-Year Strategy to Promote Health Care and Welfare for the Elderly (the New Gold Plan) that came into effect on 1 April 2000, municipalities are the insurer and the national government, prefectures and medical care insurers provide multi-layers of support to prevent excessive administrative financial burdens on the municipalities (Japan Ministry of Health, Labour and Welfare, 1999). Half of the cost of long-term care insurance administered by the Financial Stability Fund is borne by the premium payments of the insured, and the other half is funded by public funds. Of the public funds, the ratio among the national government, prefectures and local municipalities is fixed at 2:1:1. In addition, the national government contributes towards adjusting the financial gaps among municipalities because of the differences in the ratio of subscribers in their advanced age and their abilities to bear the financial burden (Japan Ministry of Health, Labour and Welfare, 2004b) and pays half of the cost for the new administrative work. To ensure impartiality between service users and non-users, in principle the users are required to pay a 10 per cent co-payment for long-term care. However, in the case of low-income elderly a maximum amount of burden is set by issuing a service fee for long-term care (ibid., 1999).

In Germany, the long-term care insurance is funded entirely by insurance contributions but only covers social care services. Health-related services continue to be covered by the separate (social) health care insurance and, similar to the UK, the boundary between the two schemes remains blurred. The funding of medical aids and medical nursing care for the elderly in residential care homes by the health care insurance in particular has been subject to controversies and adjustments (Deutscher Bundestag, 2004). Another distinct feature is that the insurance includes cash benefits which older people can use to pay informal carers (Schunk, 1998). This reflects the fact that the insurance covers only basic home care, including personal care services and household help services (Wenger, 2001). In contrast to the long-term care insurance in Japan, the insurance cover in Germany therefore is meant to be completed by either further private means or unpaid informal care.

In comparison to Japan and Germany, the Netherlands is something of a pioneer and the settledness of funding has long been high (Coolen and Weekers, 1998: 50). This is embedded in a care regime where formal care services are available universally as characteristic of the public service model. Both health and social care services are covered by a separate social insurance introduced in the late 1960s, whose forerunners go back to the mid-1950s (Knijn, 1998). The insurance covers a range of exceptional medical risks. It is compulsory for all employees (irrespective of income) and is supplemented by central government funds and out-of-pocket payments (Kerkstra, 1996). This makes for a strong element of universalism. However, concerns about expenditure, coupled with a renewed emphasis on subsidiarity and the primacy of self-help (in this case, informal care), have started to weaken the universalist orientation of the social insurance (Visser-Jansen and Knipscheer, 2004).

Estonia is an interesting case as it mixes social insurance and tax-based funding (see Kivisaar and Soots, 2006). The National Health Insurance Fund introduced in 1992 pays for home nursing services. Based on the principle of universalism, the Fund covers almost 95 per cent of the population and about 80–90 per cent of all health-related costs. This contrasts with the limited availability of services. In contrast, social care services are funded by the municipalities through taxes. Social care services comprise a wide range of domestic services as well as support in daily life. Eligibility criteria are based on the idea of subsidiarity, and access is strongly dependent on the ability of the family to provide care. Altogether this makes for a relatively low settledness of the governance through funding.

In contrast to all other countries discussed so far, the US relies extensively on private funding, which considerably undermines the settledness of funding. Until recently, public reimbursement for home care services has been minimal except for the indigent. This resonates with a care regime that is based on means testing, where political power over care services is highly decentralised and fragmented. In response to crises in funding Medicare/Medicaid, however, initiatives have been introduced to encourage people to stay at home to reduce costs (Sloane, 2005; Wilensky, 2005). The Program of All Inclusive Care for the Elderly (PACE) is an optional benefit under Medicare and Medicaid for people over 55 years of age who are frail enough to meet their state's standards for nursing home care (Centers for Medicare and Medicaid Services, 2003b). Depending on the case, Medicare and Medicaid might pay some home care costs that are related to medical care but not for informal carers. For most patients, though, the comprehensive service package permits them to continue living at home rather than be institutionalised. The PACE organisation must offer a service package that includes all Medicare and Medicaid services provided by that state as well as an additional 16 services, and in turn receives a fixed monthly payment per patient from Medicare and Medicaid. Persons enrolled in PACE may also have to pay a monthly premium, depending on their eligibility for Medicare and Medicaid. However, it is available only in the 14 states that have chosen to offer PACE under Medicaid.

Significantly, only in Sweden and the Netherlands is the funding of formal health and social care services integrated, further strengthening the settledness of governing arrangements. In Sweden, the funding of health and social care has long been separate among the county councils and the municipalities, which provided a lever for encouraging municipalities to develop community-based services. However, the restructuring of the delivery of nursing and medical health and social care services in Sweden since the 1990s was accompanied by a redefinition of the financial responsibility of the counties and the municipalities. In general, taxes paid at the council level are used to cover hospital care. The new regulations in contrast assigned the financial responsibility for hospital patients ready for discharge to the municipalities. The municipalities were also given incentives to set up a comprehensive and integrated provision of home care and to improve the cooperation between hospitals and the ambulatory sector (SOU, 2000; Landstingsförbundet, 2002). The integration of funding is even stronger in the Netherlands, where the social insurance for exceptional medical risks covers both health and social care services.

Finally, there are interesting variations in terms of the degree of decentralisation of funding arrangements, which are particularly strong in Italy but also apparent in Japan and Sweden. As the discussion above suggests, funding from sub-central sources alone does not make for the unsettledness of governing arrangements. Instead, this occurs when political power over formal care services is fragmented and lacks cohesion in terms of connections between different locales of political power. Italy is a prime example because there are not only many different schemes of funding but there is also a lack of integration between them (Polverini et al., 2004) coupled with an almost complete absence of central-level regulation (Trifiletti, 1998). A recent ruling of the Italian Constitutional Court has further strengthened the decentralisation of governing arrangements, and the national government can now no longer attach any strings to grants to regions (Ferioli, 2004). This is significant, as funds from the national level make up almost one-fifth of the social budget spent by municipalities (Ministero del Lavoro e delle Politiche Sociali, 2005).

Health services are regional, although minimum quality standards of services are set at national level and free at the point of use. Services include community services for patients unable to attend their GP practice and, where available, home nursing and rehabilitation. In contrast, municipalities organise the funding of social care services although funding comes from the regions with some financial support from the national government. The services are means tested and comprise help with personal care and housework. The unsettledness of funding makes subsidiarity real, not least as the legal obligation to provide monetary support or support in kind extends to relatives up to the second degree. Although legally this obligation can only be enforced on request by the person in need of care, many municipalities de facto try to enforce such obligations without the necessary initial request (Aimar et al., 2004; Lamura et al., 2004).

By comparison, the decentralised governing arrangements in Japan are characterised by greater cohesion and the responsibilities of local and regional levels are defined clearly, as well as embedded in the long-term care insurance as a national framework. One goal of Japan's Gold Plan was to reconstruct the vertically divided system between health and welfare services and to establish a system by which service users can receive comprehensive services from a variety of institutions of their choice. A second goal was to separate long-term care from the coverage of the health care insurance, and to establish a system which aims to decrease cases of *social hospitalisation* as the first step towards restructuring the social security system as a whole. Despite initial criticism (see Arai and Kumamoto, 2004), preliminary findings suggest that municipal delivery responsibility for comprehensive care combined with the tripartite public government funding (national, prefecture, municipality) and consumer choice is working (Matsuda, 2002; Campbell and Ikegami, 2003; Ikegami et al, 2003).

Although public funding dominates, then, the settledness of governing through funding varies widely across countries. This reflects the relative strength of ideas of universalism and means testing as embedded in different care regimes. The differences between the UK and Sweden as two countries where tax funding prevails are an indicative example. In addition, the relative integration of funding of health and social care services positively contributes to the settledness of funding (as the example of the Netherlands demonstrates) as does the cohesion of political power over formal care services (with Italy as an extreme case of fragmentation).

GOVERNING FORMAL CARE SERVICES THROUGH RULES: HIERARCHY WITH SOME PROFIT SEEKING

Governing through rules is about regulation – about coordinating the diverse actions that make up home care. This can follow a variety of principles and associated mechanisms but in relation to formal care services hierarchy (through command-and-control rules), norms (through negotiations) and profit seeking (through competition) are especially important. Hierarchy is likely to make for a particularly high degree of integration of governing through rules. Governing through rules more often than not consists of a mix of different logics, and individual countries show specific mixes of different types of rules. Such mixes are often closely linked to different aspects of the context of the governance of home care. Command-and-control rules based on hierarchy, for example, point to both a public interest in and a public capacity to govern formal care services. Ideas about the primacy of formal care services and full-time female employment as the norm, typical of the dual breadwinner/ institutional care model, are likely to strengthen the public interest in formal care. In contrast, ideas about the primacy of family care and women as housewives/part-time employees as the norm, typical of the family care model, is less conducive to promoting a public interest in formal care services. The public capacity to govern formal care service is predicated on the resources of the state and more specifically the political power over formal care services. Extensive resources of the state as an actor are likely to enhance the capacity to govern as will the relative cohesion of political power.

Historically, governing formal care services through rules has been most closely associated with the logic of associations, whereas contemporary governing arrangements largely present themselves as a combination of different types of rules (for an overview, see Table 4.5). In this respect, the prominence of hierarchy in the form of command-and-control rules is particularly striking, as is the increasing importance of profit-seeking through competition. The first aspect points to the growing integration of formal care services into the welfare state; the second reflects recent reforms concerned with the introduction of market mechanisms. The combination of different logics has conflicting effects on the relative integration of governance and the associated fragmentation in terms of locales of governance.

Especially Sweden, but also the UK, New Zealand and Estonia are examples of countries where rules based on hierarchy are strong. In all four countries, political power over formal care services is characterised by a high

Table 4.5 Rules relating to formal care services

Rules in relation to	Predominant combination of rules		
	Hierarchy/profit seeking	Norms/hierarchy	Norms/hierarchy/ profit seeking
Health care services	UK, New Zealand, Estonia (central hierarchy)	Japan	US (national Medicare); Germany (decentralised hierarchy)
Social care services	UK (central/local hierarchy); New Zealand, Estonia (local hierarchy)	Japan (local hierarchy)	Germany (decentralised hierarchy); US (local hierarchy)
Both health and social care services	Sweden (regional/ local hierarchy)		Netherlands

degree of cohesion, and the state has extensive resources even though the relative centralisation of rules based on hierarchy varies.

In Sweden, command-and-control rules are embedded in a care regime that is based on the primacy of formal care services which have long been part of the fabric of governing formal care services. This makes for not only extensive resource of governance but also the cohesion of political power over home care. Here it is indicative that formal care services were already established in the 1950s. This co-exists, however, with a high degree of decentralisation, and some observers even suggest that the large differences at local level make it more appropriate to talk about a multitude of welfare municipalities rather than a single welfare state (Trydegard and Thorslund, 2001). The term 'welfare municipalities' applies not only to the accessibility of services but also to their organisation. The Swedish municipalities enjoy considerable freedom in relation to defining the scope and the volume of services, as well as over the definition of eligibility criteria and the charges for services. This has led to unequal access to services (Trydegard, 2000, 2003). Not surprisingly the organisation of services is also characterised by diversity. In half of the localities, county councils have delegated the responsibility for home nursing to municipalities (National Board of Health and Welfare, 2000). Also the devolution of responsibility has led to the development of very different forms of cooperation to set up integrated service provision (SOU, 2000).

By contrast, in New Zealand the administration is highly centralised and health and social care services are funded through general taxation set by parliament. As a result, rules are based on a strict top-down hierarchy. Moreover, upon its return to power in 1999, the Labour government promised an integrated budget for health and social care through the Ministry of Health, thus further amalgamating the rules for social care which previously were less centralised. Similarly, in the case of the UK the strength of rules based on hierarchy is closely tied to a political system that is unitary as well as highly centralised. In the case of health care services, for example, the central government enjoys considerable control and not only fixes the annual budget of the NHS but also heads the administration of health services. Local health authorities and providers are therefore ultimately creatures of statute and depend on central government for the space in which they operate (Burau and Kröger, 2004).

Japan is the classic example where rules based on hierarchy are combined with rules based on norms. This reflects the continued strength of the notion of subsidiarity characteristic of a gender culture that has traditionally given primacy to care by the family in the first instance, and by civil society in the second instance, but which is increasingly combined with public regulation of home care. Under Japan's long-term care insurance system the central government, prefectures and municipalities are mandated to work together to implement long-term care for the elderly. While the outline of the Gold Plan is set at the national level, localities retain significant flexibility in adapting it to local norms. Interestingly, this policy introduced a new concept to Japanese society that long-term care is no longer expected from the family or allocated by the state on the basis of need but rather a social contract based on a system of mandatory contributions, uniform entitlements and consumer choice (Izuhara, 2003). This redefines care of the elderly from a filial to a social function and as such represents a radical departure from the traditional gender culture based on the primacy of the family.

The picture is more complicated in the remaining countries where rules based on profit seeking also play an important role. The Netherlands is characterised by an interesting mix of different types of rules. The logic of associations, together with the logic of the state, has long been strong and this is embedded in a gender culture that combines ideas of subsidiarity, especially relating to the involvement of civil society in formal care services and of universality that family care needs to be supported by formal care services to a considerable extent. The still dominant private non-profit providers have their origins in earlier denominational organisations, but gradually have became integrated into the public care regime (Knijn, 1998). Together with the insurance funds and professional organisations, they make up the Health Insurance Council. This is a statutory non-public body that the government has to consult with and that also oversees the running of the health insurance. Nevertheless, central government enjoys a considerable influence and sets the overall budgetary framework, quality standards and criteria for the allocation of services (Österle, 2001). Since the early 1990s, the logic of the market has been added, especially in the form of *regulated competition*. This seems to have considerably upset the balance between existing logics and introduced a high level of conflict (Knijn, 1998).

The same is true for Germany, where the introduction of the long-term care insurance in 1995/96 opened up the care sector for private for-profit providers on equal terms with the non-profit providers that traditionally dominated this sector. The corresponding set of regulations, however, reflects a complex mixture of rules based on hierarchy and profit seeking. The for-profit/non-profit providers' associations and the long-term care insurance funds negotiate the contents and price of care packages at state level. The home care sector therefore presents itself as a highly regulated market with only limited opportunities for service providers to set prices and define care packages. In contrast, rules of profit seeking prevail in relation to personnel, where the for-profit providers in particular try to cut costs (Theobald, 2004).

Rules in the form of competition through profit seeking are much more influential in the US. Indeed the major impetus for moves towards more emphasis on home care in the US is a financial one, the promise that home care will save money! Ironically, in part because of the rapid rise of a for-profit market in home care, concerns have been raised about the increasing Medicare expenditures for home care. Reflecting this concern over rising costs, a prospective payment system (PPS) for home health care was implemented in 2000 which requires home health care agencies to ensure efficient service delivery by monitoring the cost of care and the number of home health visits (Gundling, 2000)

Unlike the countries discussed so far, it is difficult to place Italy. This reflects considerable variations between regions: the rules in the most dynamic regions like Lombardy are now close to the hierarchy/profit-seeking type, while other regions such as those in the South are more static and characterised by a mix of rules based on norms and hierarchy. Yet other regions find themselves in an intermediate position combining rules based on norms, hierarchy and profit seeking (Da Roit, 2005).

As in the case of funding, divisions between central, regional and local levels of governing came into play in relation to rules. Sub-central levels are particularly important in relation to social care services, reflecting the historical development of such services and their traditionally marginal role in welfare services. For example, under the US Constitution the states not the federal government have primary responsibility for the health and welfare of their populations. While in reality Washington has significant influence in health and welfare policy because of its vast resources particularly over health care for those over age 65, under Medicare the states retain considerable control. As a result there remains significant variation in services across states and localities, despite federal initiatives over the years. This is even more the case in social welfare, where there is no national policy. Because of the multi-faceted nature of home care, there is little consistency from one sub-central level to the next in the US. This fragmentation is reinforced by the heavy emphasis on the private sector in many areas surrounding home care.

At the same time there are also examples where such local hierarchies are increasingly complemented by central hierarchies. The long-term care insurance in Germany, for example, supports federal regulation of access and benefits in the case of care dependency, whereas the responsibility for the implementation of the long-term care insurance has been reassigned from the municipalities to the states. Importantly, the law also defines the responsibilities of states, municipalities, insurance funds and service providers for developing an adequate infrastructure. This makes for a relatively tight integrated system of decentralised responsibility. Similarly, in the UK the welfare mix and privatisation policies have further increased the traditional variations across different localities, but have also made them more visible. This has been taken up by recent reforms. A new regulatory body is mandated to define standards and assess attainment. This is complemented by the

Institute for Excellence which gives guidance on good practice. Indeed, Johnson (2001) suggests that the continued commitment to decentralisation is now combined with more central government surveillance and control, thus limiting the autonomy of local authorities and local providers.

In summary, governing through rules is characterised by hybrids that centre around the rules based on hierarchy and that often include elements of profit seeking. The relative importance of hierarchy and its specific combinations with other logics reflect different degrees of public interest in home care, together with different capacities for governing. For example, while rules based on hierarchy exist in both Sweden and the US, they are stronger in Sweden, resonating with a care regime based on the public service model and political power over formal care services that is cohesive.

DISCUSSION AND CASE STUDIES

Across our countries the governance of formal care services through delivery, funding and rules is characterised by more or less fragmentation. Variations exist relating to the degree and the type of fragmentation. The two are closely related: the types of fragmentation mirror divisions between public and private responsibilities, between levels of governing, as well as between health and social care services. Public provision, integration of health and social care services and integration of different levels of governing are all conducive to integrated governing arrangements. The different types of fragmentation also closely mirror the context of governing: gender cultures and care regimes offer more or less favourable conditions for public provision, and the relative cohesion (and partly centralisation) of political power facilitates more or less strong integration between different levels of governing. Formal care services are therefore an area of governance that highlights the importance of the salient divisions between public and private and between national and local levels. The characteristics of gender cultures and care regimes help clarify the relative strength of public–private divisions, while the characteristics of political power over care helps us understand the relative strength of national–local divisions.

The following case studies analyse in more detail the specific interplay between ideas and institutions in relation to the reform of formal care services. Japan is an example of increased integration, especially in terms of funding and rules, while developments in Sweden point in the opposite direction. In both cases, however, the changes cannot easily be predicted from the contextual factors underpinning the governance of home care, and instead point to a dynamic and highly specific interplay between ideas and institutions which also provides a platform for interactions between state and non-state actors. In Japan, the emergence of new actors that succeeded building coalitions with inside actors is key, while in Sweden the existence of distinct levels of politics (at national and local levels) provides an important lever for change.

Japan's Long-term Insurance and Changing Welfare Politics

From the outside, Japan's adoption of its long-term insurance with its provision of comprehensive coverage for home care is surprising. One might expect that a country with a traditional filial culture of care for the elderly would be among the last to embrace the idea that the government should have a central role in funding (and regulating) home care. However, societal changes, together with problem pressures, have meant that ideas about the relative support of the state, especially of formal care services, have started to change.

But Japan also has a pragmatic policy history, and by the mid-1990s pressure was building for concerted governmental action to deal with the problems emerging from the confluence of demographic and social forces. A combination of the world's highest longevity and a decline in fertility accelerated the speed of societal ageing, with those over 65 predicted to account for 25 per cent of the total population by 2015 (Campbell and Ikegami, 2003). Complicating these demographic trends is a shift in the structure and function of Japanese families. In terms of structure, there has been a dramatic shift towards independent living and in the number of elderly-only households. Moreover, the pool of family carers is shrinking, partly because of women joining the labour market for paid work, which is increasingly necessary for household survival. Adding to these demographic and social changes, the end of the economic boom and the subsequent recession led to a decline in tax revenue, making it increasingly difficult for the government to match the expected increase in social security expenditure of an ageing society.

Growing deficits in medical insurance were especially problematic in Japan, partly due to the fact that most institutional long-term care has been provided in hospitals (Izuhara, 2003). In contrast to the social welfare sector, health care costs were not capped by budget but left open ended. As a result, the number of elderly inpatients increased tenfold from 1973 to 1993 (Ikegami et al., 2003). The inappropriate and expensive social admissions to hospitals and the inadequate supply of home care under social welfare were seen as an urgent problem in the light of the trends above.

In response, the Liberal Democratic Party produced the Gold Plan in 1989 as its major campaign promise for the Lower House election early the next year, following a major defeat in an Upper House election. The Gold Plan is a first indication of increased state support and as such also marks the beginning of a change of the care regime. The Gold Plan, formally called the Ten-Year Strategy to Promote Health and Welfare for the Aged, set targets for a major expansion of services. The Gold Plan was implemented and further expanded in 1994 to the New Gold Plan (ibid.). Despite these changes, however, serious problems were emerging. On the one hand, this system was expensive at a time when the Japanese electorate was seen as opposed to tax increases. On the other, the administrative apparatus for deciding eligibility and providing services was still essentially the same as that for public assistance, and unsuited for large-scale services to many people. These and other considerations, including the fragmentation of health and welfare services, a general anti-bureaucratic mood, and a corresponding interest in consumerism and market-based solutions, brought a search for a new approach. In essence, Japan turned from the road to Scandinavia and opted instead for a social insurance model somewhat similar to that initiated in Germany in 1995 (Cuellar and Wiener, 2000).

The accumulated pressures provided a window of opportunity for change that was strengthened by extensive lobbying from outside, together with an alliance with resourceful actors from within that made for a strong coalition for reform. Japan's experience with long-term care insurance (LTCI) is an interesting case of a shift from insider to outsider politics. For Eto (2001), in fact, it was an issue 'outside the established political system' where the conventional policy community of social welfare was destabilised, thereby allowing non-established political players to emerge. Typically the process for formulating Japanese welfare policy begins with welfare ministry bureaucrats drafting a bill and forwarding it to the appropriate advisory council to allocate benefits among interested groups (ibid.: 33–4). After council approval, the bill is sent to the ruling party caucus and then presented to the full Diet (parliament).

The advisory council in charge of welfare for elderly people is the Council on Health and Welfare for the Elderly which largely reflected the views of those who resisted change to the LTCI, specifically local officials who were exempt from responsibility for managing the welfare system and representatives of those on a low income who did not own their homes or have relatives to take care of them, and who could pass a government means test. On the other side were emerging forces who demanded a more open process which acknowledged the failure of existing policy to address the problem of caring for the middle-class elderly. During the process of drafting reform, new political players, including ordinary citizens and mayors of small-scale municipal governments, emerged as important players. As a result, these outsider groups became actively involved in the political process and shifted from being simple watchers of 'the political game being played by the "professional" actors, politicians and media representatives' (Hrebenar et al., 1998: 551) to being actors themselves.

By the late 1980s, taking care of the disabled elderly was a problem that could no longer be solved by families on their own. In Japanese society where, according to the traditional gender division of labour, 'the man goes to work and the woman is at home', caring for the elderly has usually been carried out by women (Japan Ministry of Health, Labour and Welfare, 1999: 39). Faced with a situation where they were forced to resign from work and/or give up their lives outside the home entirely, women became active. With the creation of the Women's Association for Improving an Ageing Society (the Women's Association) in 1986 came an advocacy force for socialising care, the idea that care of the elderly should not be left to the family only but should be supported by the entire society. In the mid-1990s, the Women's Association was joined by a new citizen action group (the Citizens' Committee) that championed approval of the LTCI. In 1996, influential Japanese who were worried about the LTCI bill's dimming prospects urged the Diet to approve the legislation. They were infuriated because the government had not responded to public demands to socialise care for the elderly, reflected in polls showing that over 75 per cent of the public wanted an LTCI system (Eto, 2001). In response to official inaction, they organised a citizens' action group, the Ten Thousand Citizens' Committee to Realise a Public Care of the Elderly System (Citizens' Committee). With the hope of informing parliamentary deliberations, the Citizens' Committee proposed a Citizens' Amendment. The Committee organised a working team composed of experts and researchers in related fields. Although only a few of the proposals of the Citizens' Committee were incorporated into the LTCI law, this was the first time that voters succeeded in having part of a bill revised (ibid.).

Municipal leaders, particularly the mayors of towns and villages, were hesitant to assume responsibility for managing the new system and came out against it. Consequently the public began to suspect that all mayors were opposed to the LTCI system, despite their key role in implementing it. In order to counter this negative image, 81 mayors established the Mayors' Association to Promote Welfare Administration for their Residents (Welfare Mayors) in November 1997. They supported the LTCI system, believing that it would provide them with a good opportunity to promote municipal welfare policy and demonstrate their leadership. Their stance stood in strong contrast to that of mayors opposed to the LTCI system. Even after it became law on 9 December 1997, the negative mayors' group demanded that the government act to change the law's provisions. In cooperation with the Women's Association and the Citizens' Committee, and through effective use of the mass media, core members of the Welfare Mayors were able to protect LTCI from the forces that intended to derail it (ibid.).

With the adoption of the LTCI, the funding for long-term care became unified both at the central level and at the point of service delivery. With their entitled amount, individuals are free to choose among the agencies or facilities and the service mix of health and social services in community care (Ikegami et al., 2003). Under the LTCI, long-term care has become part of a social contract based upon a system of mandatory contributions, uniform entitlements and consumer choice. According to Izuhara (2003), this contribution is an integral part of the new social contract and the principle of social justice is defined as 'everybody contributes'. One of the LTCI's aims is to remove the stigma attached to the traditional notion of means-tested social welfare, and the contractual nature of the scheme is emphasised: the use of services is based on the contract signed by two parties (service users and providers) in an equal relationship (Ikegami and Campbell, 2002). As part of the wider socialisation of care provision, a quasi-market approach was introduced. In order to balance the division between home and institutional care, locally based groups and organisations have emerged to provide a range of welfare services. Although only approved organisations can provide services, non-profit and for-profit organisations are encouraged to do so. Overall, then, the LTCI not only changed the way home care is financed, provided and ruled but also has had a significant impact on gender roles and the relationship between family and government responsibility.

Challenging Service Provision in the Context of Multi-level Politics in Sweden

In Sweden, public home help services for the elderly were established in the 1950s and expanded during the 1960s and 1970s. Since the 1980s, and in particular the 1990s, a decrease in the proportion among the elderly receiving services can be found. Care policies are defined basically at the national level, but the municipalities enjoy considerable freedom when implementing national goals. In the following discussion, the reduction of home help services is analysed against the background of the development of changing care policies at the national level and its implementation at the local level. The overall idea of public responsibility for elderly care services has remained unchanged but the reductions can be explained by ambitious national policies implemented under cost containment, by national laws only specifying basic goals, by the freedom of the municipality to decide on the measures on its own and by changing ideas on the elderly and the ageing process.

Public home help services for older people began in the 1950s and quickly advanced to become an important part of the Swedish universal welfare state. The access to social services became a social right for all citizens based on needs, and was therefore to be paid for and organised by society (Gough,

1994). Even the changing gender relations since the 1960s pushed the expansion of home help services. Care services enable the simultaneous participation in paid and unpaid work for both women and men. In rural areas, more specific care services for the elderly could close the care gap that had emerged because of the migration of women from the rural areas to the cities (Hirdman, 1990; Brodin, 2005).

In the 1960s and 1970s, the public elderly care services expanded, peaking in the 1970s when more than 30 per cent of the population aged 65 years and above received services mainly delivered at home (Brodin, 2005). Home help for the elderly was only loosely regulated within the Social Help Act, and thus home help services expanded more or less without any regulation. Parallel to the introduction of the Social Help Act in the 1960s, the Social Commission was set up to analyse the public responsibility for care of the elderly and the disabled. The report of the Social Commission provided the basis for the Social Service Act, which came into effect in 1982 and is still the legislative basis for the delivery of home-based services for the elderly.

In its report, the Social Commission described the statutory responsibilities of the municipalities for services in different areas, including the delivery of different types of social services and structural measures aimed at good planning. With the suggestions the Social Commission took on ideas that the New Left had been arguing for, notably for care services to be oriented towards the social model of community care. Within the area of elderly care, the Social Commission confirmed the idea of public responsibility and at the same time emphasised the importance of individual self-determination of the elderly. The Social Commission saw only a limited need for regulation in the area of elderly care, and argued that only general goals should be specified.

The liberal social minister of the conservative–liberal government agreed with the report but made two changes. He highlighted the need for a more active role of the elderly, who should be viewed as more healthy and independent. In addition, he emphasised the need for a more active role of the civil organisations in service provision, in particular with regard to social integration. Nearly all organisations that were asked to give evidence were supportive of the proposals. The national organisation of the municipalities emphasised that the law provided only general guidelines that leave room for self-government. The pensioners' organisations for their part expected an expansion of services. However, the opposite was true. The law required a reallocation of resources within municipalities and there was no additional support available from the national government. The elderly care policies in the 1980s were therefore characterised by the dilemma that care services should be developed further, but under the condition of cost containment. The idea of healthy ageing and of more autonomous elderly seemed to present a solution to the dilemma. Care services should offer help aimed at self-help, and traditional housework should be replaced by tasks promoting rehabilitation and an active participation of the elderly in social life (Szebehely, 1995, 1996). Despite the ambitious goals of the law the proportion of the elderly receiving services decreased, in particular in relation to housework duties (Szebehely, 2000).

Due the general nature of the Social Service Act a parliamentary committee, the Eldercare Working Committee, was assembled to evaluate the development (see Brodin, 2005) and the proposals of the committee provided the basis for a new law. According to the committee's report, the law should focus on preventive health measures to promote healthy ageing, open up service provision to private entrepreneurs and civil organisations with regard to housework and social activities, and initiate the de-hospitalisation of care for the elderly under a unified public responsibility by the municipalities. The social-democratic social minister explained that, similar to the Social Service Act, the municipalities and county councils could not count on additional funds from the national government to support the implementation of the bill.

When the bill was passed, a parliamentary commission, the Ädel Commission, was set up to outline suggestions for the re-regulation and reorganisation of elderly care services under the leadership of the municipalities. According to the committee, the dual responsibility of county councils and municipalities had led to public elderly care being dominated by a medical rather than a social model. Instead, the commission suggested that the municipalities should take on the entire statutory responsibility for all forms of public elderly care. The nursing homes should be transferred from the county councils to the municipalities and integrated into the municipalities' special forms of accommodation. The municipalities should receive the county councils' financial resources related to the nursing homes. In addition, the municipalities should take on the responsibility for all medical services relating to the elderly, excluding medical treatment provided by doctors. And finally, the municipalities had to offer adequate home-based care for hospital patients ready for discharge, or were obliged to pay the costs for the hospital stay. The responsibility for the implementation of the reform was given to the municipalities and county councils. The economic framework, a better allocation of resources, was based on the principle of local self-government.

The reform, which came into effect in 1992, was criticised by the parliamentary Social Committee because it did not give the municipalities enough freedom to private providers. The conservative–liberal government which followed the social-democratic government passed a bill to increase such possibilities. In addition, due to the different regulations of fees in the municipalities and county councils a unified regulation of fees was seen as necessary. However, the conservative–liberal government limited the public regulation of fees and the new sets of rules, which came into effect in 1993, required only that fees should be reasonable. As such, the fees should not exceed the costs for the municipalities and should leave the individual with an income for basic personal needs (Feltenius, 2004).

Neither the Ädel Reform nor the opening up of service delivery for private providers changed the public financial responsibility for elderly care provision. However, during the 1990s the number of elderly people receiving services fell dramatically. The home help services increasingly concentrated on frail elderly people while those requiring merely basic household service often no longer qualified for home help services. In addition to stricter regulations, the increasing fees for home help services resulted in a withdrawal of potential care recipients (Trydegard, 2003; Szebehely, 1999a,b, 2000). The changing patterns of care provision were strongly related to the Ädel Reform. The financial incentive for the municipalities to offer home-based care for discharged hospital patients resulted in an increase of care provision to frail elderly people at home. However, the development was strengthened due to demographic change, with a rising proportion of elderly people over 80 years in the population in the 1990s, but the demand was not met with adequate financial resources (Palme, et al., 2002; Trydegard, 2003).

The possibility for the municipalities to restrict elderly care services in a time of financial constraints is related to regulations in the Social Service Act (see Rauch, 2005). Social services entitlements are defined as individual rights but the character of an individual right is weakened in two respects. The content and volume of care rights are unspecified and the only requirement is that the individual has a reasonable standard of living and that public support supports independent living. Furthermore, public social care services should be granted on the condition that the needs cannot be met in other ways. Due to this definition of entitlements, it is unclear whether access to potential family care or sufficient financial means could be defined as 'other ways'. Moreover, the municipalities enjoy freedom to regulate the fees on their own, with only weak constraints from the national government.

The increasing differences among the municipalities with regard to the level of fees and the often low definition of a basic income for personal needs were a central criticism in the final evaluation of the development of care services by the National Board of Health and Welfare following the Ädel Reform (as quoted in Brodin, 2005). After an inquiry into the regulation of fees in 2002, Parliament passed an act defining maximum fees and a basic income for personal needs (Feltenius, 2004). Further signs of re-regulations at the national level can be seen in the proposed National Development Plan for Care for the Elderly. Among other things, the plan suggests that on the basis of a further inquiry the need for more specified regulations should be analysed (Ministry of Health and Social Affairs, 2006).

5. Integrating informal care provision

Until the 1980s, informal care delivery was a neglected area in mainstream social policy and scientific debate in most Western countries, despite its importance for care provision. Expectations of a gap in informal family care provision due to demographic and social changes as well as research findings on the significance of informal care opened up the social–political debate for the issue (Hochschild, 1995). The increasing recognition of informal care delivery is reflected in the introduction of new types of cash payments to support informal care giving, and a new balance between the provision of in-kind services and payments. Daly and Lewis (2000a) describe this new balance between cash payments and services as a crucial trend in the area of social care where the mixture differs among and within welfare states: 'It involves not just the old either/or constellation of service, cash transfer or taxation but rather differentiation in the manner in which cash and services are combined to support private or public care on the part of the welfare states' (ibid.: 292). As a result, the boundary between formal care provided by public, private for-profit or non-profit organisations and informal care provided by family members, relatives, friends or neighbours has become an area of conflict and re-negotiation as well as newly developed forms of cooperation.

The restructurings centre on the macro level related to new forms of governance of care provision but also have implications for the micro level of daily care giving (Daly and Lewis, 1998). Care provision following the family logic based on kinship, moral and personal obligations has to be combined mainly with elements of the state logic, with its emphasis on laws and hierarchy, but also with those of market logic, characterised by the principles of competition and freedom of choice for the users. The measures introduced define how and the degree to which informal care traditionally provided within the family framework has become formalised and integrated into the public sphere. The different types of support of informal care work, the modes and level of funding and the rules or regulations set up are decisive for the degree and form of integration.

Within the context of home care governance, the analysis of governance of informal care elucidates the process of integration of informal care delivery in the overall provision of home care. It contributes to the understanding of home care governing in several ways. First, the analysis of the different measures introduced specifies ways and degrees of the integration of informal care in overall care provision. It reveals the embeddedness of the process within the care regimes and the policy subsystems in the countries compared. The orientation of the care regimes, towards the family on the one hand and a care provision based on universalism or means testing on the other, as well as the interplay of national and local levels are decisive for the development of different measures and thus for the mode of integration. Second, the analysis shows the ways in which different logics, in particular the family and the state, are combined, and reveals that in countries with an emphasis on the family logic in policy development, the formalisation of informal care work is impeded. Third, the analysis shows the actors involved in the process with the state as a key actor and its interplay with further societal actors and movements such as the disabled people's movement or carers' organisations.

The analysis here consists of three parts. First, the focus on the governance of delivery of care aims to reveal the different support strategies in home-based care provision in the nine countries. Second, the mode and level of funding related to different types of cash payments for informal care giving are analysed, illustrating the different societal sectors (state, market, voluntary) involved and the consequences for the social situation of informal care giving. Third, the discussion clarifies the changing regulations within certain defined areas of informal care that in addition to funding can be viewed as significant starting-points for a more formalised care provision. The analysis proceeds from the assumption that the care regimes, in particular their predominant strategy to support home care, are decisive for the measures introduced, their mode and level of funding, and the rules set up. Despite the highly gendered area of informal care giving, the weak position of female actors in the process of policy development makes for a contradictory influence of the ideas related to the gender culture, which range from a neglect of the interests of women to a consideration of their family or employment situation until an active participation of female actors in the public debate and policy development is evident.

GOVERNING INFORMAL CARE THROUGH DELIVERY: THE EMBEDDEDNESS OF SUPPORT STRATEGIES

In most Western countries, a variety of measures have been established to support home care. The approaches in different countries can be distinguished primarily according to their emphasis on support via formal care provision provided by public, private for-profit and non-profit providers, or via economic support for informal care giving within the family framework. The governance of formal care services includes different societal sectors (state, market and voluntary) while the state or state-related actors at national or local levels are solely involved in the provision of economic support.

Support strategies for home care provision are developing, embedded in the definition of public, private or family responsibility for care related to the care regimes and the corresponding policy subsystem in the area with its interplay of the national and local levels. The relationship to ideas on gender relations, notably on female labour market participation, is much more incongruous, although in these countries, care provision within the family framework is conducted mainly by wives or daughters. Patterns of informal care provision differ, however, and are influenced by the selected support strategy. In Table 5.1, the support strategies, their embeddedness in different care regimes and the patterns of formal and informal care provision are mapped out in a cross-country comparison.

Table 5.1 Support strategy and care regimes

	Public service model	Means-tested model	Subsidiarity model	Family care model
Formal care	*Predominant* Sweden Netherlands Japan	*Predominant* US New Zealand UK	*Predominant* Japan	*Predominant* –
	Secondary –	*Secondary* –	*Secondary* Germany	*Secondary* Italy Estonia
Economic support for informal care giving	*Predominant* –	*Predominant* –	*Predominant* Germany	*Predominant* Estonia Italy
	Secondary Sweden Netherlands	*Secondary* UK	*Secondary* Japan	*Secondary* –

In Table 5.1, the countries are organised according to their prevalent support strategy related to home-based care, oriented towards either economic support for informal care via cash payments or the provision of formal care services. The table also shows the strong relationship between the care regimes and the predominant support strategy. For countries assigned to the public service and the means-tested models, the formal care provision is the predominant support strategy, while countries emphasising family care prefer cash payments related to informal care giving. Japan and Germany, the two countries oriented towards the principle of subsidiarity, have chosen two different support strategies. This can be explained by the different orientations of the long-term care insurance (LTCI) introduced in both countries since the mid-1990s. While in Japan the emphasis on support via formal care provision aims to defamilialise care provision for the frail elderly, in Germany the preference of cash payments is meant to maintain informal family care (see below).

Only in the US and New Zealand have no cash payments been introduced related to informal care provision, and the delivery of formal care services remains the only support strategy. Both countries are traditionally characterised by an emphasis on public responsibility to the needy only, and a considerable reliance on care provision privately paid or based on charity. In the US, publicly supported home care services are available within the Medicare programme, which delivers home health care to the elderly. Within Medicaid, a tax-based system, after means testing only the elderly with a very low income receive social services at home. Home care provision is dominated by family care complemented by privately paid services or private long-term care insurance. Over 75 per cent of primary care givers are women, of which 36 per cent are adult children and 40 per cent spouses with an average age of 60. The majority of primary informal care givers do not hold paying jobs, either because they are retired or because they belonged to a generation of women not in the paid workforce. Among the third who are in the labour force, about two-thirds work full time (American Society on Aging, 2006; Family Caregiver Alliance, 2006).

In New Zealand, since the 1990s, under the national ageing in place programme, home care services are increasingly publicly subsidised and gradually different types of home care are becoming universally available without charge. This reflects a gradual departure from the traditional means-tested care regime. The strategy aims at enabling the elderly to stay at home and thus to avoid more costly institutionalised care. Despite the expansion of public funding and the provision of home care services, care in the home relies considerably on informal care provided mainly by family members. The high care burden of women has become an issue in the debate. In contrast to the US, the vast majority of these carers are between 30 and 54 years of age but they are overwhelmingly female (Statistics New Zealand, 2003).

While in New Zealand a gradual change to a more universal-oriented care regime is visible, in Japan with the introduction of the LTCI a rapid change of the care regime can be found (see Chapter 4, case study on Japan). The LTCI introduced in 2001 on a national level provides the basis for the public funding of universally available long-term care services for the elderly. In setting up its LTCI, Japan opted for a social insurance model similar to that initiated in Germany in 1995, but rejected the idea of giving beneficiaries the freedom of choice between formal care provision and a cash benefit to organise necessary care privately within the family framework (Cuellar and Wiener, 2000). There appear to be three main reasons why a cash benefit was not included despite considerable debate: first, there was a desire among women to break old family patterns which cash benefits were seen as perpetuating; second, the government wanted to gradually expand long-term care (LTC) services and believed that the demand for cash benefits would overwhelm the system; and third, the aim of the reforms was to expand the infrastructure of LTC and cash benefits were seen as hampering that process (Karlsson et al., 2004: 28).

However, the issue of whether or not the LTCI should pay family carers remains an acrimonious and divisive one. The payment of cash benefits has support from a variety of women's and other groups, such as the Women's Association for Improving an Ageing Society, but opposition by others on a variety of cultural and economic grounds. The municipalities are enabled to introduce a limited Allowance for Families Caring for Elderly with a subsidy from the central government, but to date few municipalities have opted to introduce it. Only very low-income families caring for an elderly person with the severest level of care needs who are not receiving support from the LTCI are eligible, and so far only a small number of families receive this allowance (OECD, 2005b). Based on cultural traditions, daughters-in-law comprise the largest proportion of informal carers, about 35 per cent of the total, followed by husbands and wives at 27 per cent. Over 80 per cent of the total care givers are female (Japan Ministry of Health, Labour and Welfare, 2002). However, recently many women have advanced into the workplace and it became a shared understanding that it is unfair to impose the heavier burden of family care giving on women.

In Sweden and the Netherlands, a universal-oriented public service model is already well established. In Sweden, the emphasis on a public responsibility for home care for the elderly emerged in the 1950s with the gradual definition of social services for the elderly as universally available based on a citizenship right (Gough, 1994; Johansson, 1997). Furthermore, from the 1960s on, changing gender relations emphasising a dual breadwinner model pushed the expansion of social care service provision for the elderly (Hirdman, 1990). In contrast, informal care provision is defined as voluntary for the family members and as a complement to formal care provision. In 2004, 7 per cent of the population aged 65 years and older received social care funded publicly by the municipalities, compared to approximately 0.5 per cent who receive economic support for informal care giving, thus showing clearly that formal care provision is the predominant support strategy (SOS, 2005a).

Parallel to the expansion of social care provision for the elderly, two types of cash payments were introduced to support informal care giving (see Johansson, 2004; Sand, 2005; Szebehely, 2005). First, the Attendance Allowance established in the 1940s to take care of frail family members was expanded to include long-term care for frail elderly. Second, the employment of a relative by the municipalities to take care of a frail elderly person gradually emerged at the local level. Both types are optional for the municipalities; today only 63 per cent of the municipalities offer at least one of the programmes and the proportion of the elderly benefiting is negligible (Johansson, 2004). In the current debate, the increase of funds to support informal care provision economically is viewed as a risk that may lead to a reduction of resources within formal care provision, thus strengthening the care burden of informal carers and impeding female labour market participation. Instead of extending economic support for informal care giving, a leave scheme has been introduced to facilitate the combination of care for terminally ill relatives and employment responsibilities (Szebehely, 2005). The decision reflects the provision of formal care as a well-established strategy to support female labour market participation and thus the dual breadwinner model.

A third type of benefit is based on the Law of Support and Service to Disabled People of 1994, which offers different types of support to people with severe functional impairment, including the right to employ a relative as a personal assistant. The introduction of the law is strongly related to the disabled people's movement and aims to provide the opportunity to organise care and support freely. It is not primarily meant to be a programme to support informal carers (Edebalk and Svensson, 2005; Szebehely, 2005).

Despite the emphasis on the dual breadwinner model, informal care is still provided mainly by female family members dominated by spouses, wives and only to some extent husbands, as the main informal carers. In addition, the gainfully employed daughters are the main family carers of the widows or widowers and further support their fathers in taking care of their mothers (ibid.). Care services are getting involved with increasing care dependency and oriented to the elderly living on their own. Due to restructurings within care services, family carers are left with a rising responsibility, notably for housekeeping services (Trydegard, 2003; Szebehely, 2005).

In the Netherlands since the 1960s, care provision for the elderly has been defined as a public responsibility and funded by the National (Social) Insurance for Exceptional Medical Risks. A well-functioning health service is defined as a constitutional right for all inhabitants (Visser-Janssen and Knipscheer, 2004). With 7.9 per cent of the elderly aged 65 years and older receiving home care, the level compared to most of the countries selected is high (Lundsgaard, 2004a). In the Netherlands there is no law on the rights and obligations of family carers, but there is a strong tradition of informal care based on the idea of subsidiarity, which has been supported by the predominance of part-time employment among women (Pijl, 2003; European Commission, 2005). During a needs assessment, the informal care resources are taken into account and the assessor distinguishes between normal or usual care and extra care, that is, informal care (Visser-Janssen and Knipscheer, 2004). The increasing share of informal care provision defined during the assessments raises criticism and a lot of debate among care receivers, informal carers and other interest organisations to protect their rights (ibid.). Also in the Netherlands, leave schemes have been established to take care on a short-term basis in the case of an emergency to promote the combination of paid (part-time) employment and caring responsibilities (Pijl, 2003). Daughters are the main informal carers, which is facilitated by part-time employment (Visser-Janssen and Knipscheer, 2004).

The introduction of a personal budget (a cash benefit) in 1995 provided care receivers with the opportunity to establish their own care provision based on formal and informal care, including the right to employ a family member. In 2003, only 0.8 per cent of the elderly aged 65 years and older used care budgets for their care provision (Lundsgaard, 2004a). It has been a part of care service reforms in the 1990s aimed at introducing more market elements, especially choice, into health care. The notions of autonomy and independence also resonated with the critique of the self-help movement against paternalistic service provision, while the carers' organisations vote for care budgets as an opportunity to compensate informal care giving (Tjadens and Duijnstee, 2000; Kremer, 2005).

In the UK, the provision of formal care services is the prevailing strategy for supporting home care, but the provision of social care is based on means testing, meaning that only applicants on a low income receive publicly financed social care (Baldock, 2003). Since the early 1990s, government policies have acknowledged the contribution of informal carers to care arrangements. However, additional resources for or even substantive rights to support did not follow this acknowledgement in principle. Basically two types of cash payment for informal carers are available. The Invalid Care Allowance has existed since the 1970s and is the main cash benefit. It is a benefit that is paid to carers to provide them with a symbolic compensation for the loss of income due to caring activities (Pijl, 2003). In addition, the 2000 Carers' Act gave local authorities the possibility of introducing direct payments for carers. These cash payments allow employment of relatives who do not live with the person in need of care, but it is actually meant to be a support strategy for informal care provision.

Pickard (2001), following Twigg's typology (1989) of different supports for carers, states that the government policies have sought to support existing care arrangements through supporting informal carers as co-workers. The co-worker approach treats informal carers first and foremost in an instrumental way. Carers are a resource and the social care system needs to provide support only in the case of informal carers being unable to maintain their role. Informal care arrangements continue to be characterised by a predominance of female family carers, mainly children or grandchildren and more rarely spouses (Maher and Green, 2002).

Germany, Italy and Estonia represent three countries that prefer economic support for informal care provision as the dominant strategy related to the significance of family care within the logic of the family, emphasising social obligations and social relations. In Germany, until the 1990s, this was based on the principle of subsidiarity, the idea of shared responsibility for social care (mainly elderly care) between the family and society. Frail elderly people were mainly cared for by the female family members. The changing ageing structure and the growing female employment with its expected reduction of informal networks challenged the future of the model. In 1995/96, the LTCI was introduced, aimed at providing a sound financial basis for the increasing care needs. The beneficiaries were given the freedom of choice among cash benefits, enabling them to organise the care themselves, or to opt for care services. The introduction of cash benefits was meant to maintain informal care by the family and wider network while the provision of in-kind services should enable the care insurance funds responsible for the funding to control care quality (Meyer, 1996). Despite the freedom of choice, approximately 70 per cent of beneficiaries receiving care at home choose cash benefits. In 2003, 4.6 per cent of the elderly aged 65 years and older received cash benefits only, 1.1 per cent a combination of cash benefits and services, and 2.3 per cent opted for formal home care services only (Federal Statistical Office, 2005d). Informal care provision is still provided mainly by female family members (73 per cent) primarily wives and daughters. Sixty per cent of the main informal carers are aged 55 years or older. Of the informal carers between 15 and 64 years, 60 per cent are not gainfully employed while only 19 per cent are working full time (Giese and Wiegel, 2000; Schneekloth and Leven, 2003). This reflects the notably low labour market participation of women in the age group over 55 years (European Commission, 2005).

Italy has been described in the literature as the family care model where the responsibility for care provision is delegated to the family (see Bettio and Plantenga, 2004). While formal care provision is still limited, there is an increasing monetary transfer aimed at supporting informal care provision within the family framework. Three different types of cash payment can be distinguished. While on a national level state disability pensions and state care allowances have been introduced to improve living conditions of the disabled elderly and to enable them to stay with their families, since the 1990s at a local level additional care allowances have been introduced by municipalities or regions (Lamura et al., 2001). The different payments have not been developed in an integrated approach but instead a fragmented structure can be seen, which can be viewed as a development by default rather than by design. The development reflects the highly decentralised and even fragmented policy subsystem characteristic of the Italian approach to support home care.

Nevertheless, societal structures are changing, with fewer women prepared and/or being able to provide informal care. According to the EUROFAMCARE study, which represents the only nationwide study on primary family carers in Italy so far, the great majority of primary family carers are children, mainly daughters or daughters-in-law (56.8 per cent) followed by spouses, mainly wives (10.9 per cent). Informal carers are largely concentrated in the 45–64-year-old age group and 43 per cent are employed (Quattrini, 2006). This raises the need for policies aimed at enhancing the conciliation between professional duties and caring responsibilities. In a situation of a lack of alternatives, migrant care workers coming to Italy now provide a considerable share of the informal care (Polverini and Lamura, 2004).

In Estonia, since the independence from the Soviet Union, health care and long-term care policies have changed dramatically (Saks et al., 2003). Different types of home care provision have been introduced, including social and home-nursing care, but the availability is still limited (see Kivisaar and Soots, 2006). In addition, a Caregiver Allowance in the form of a cash benefit as the basis for self-organised care has been established. Defined on a national level, the Caregiver Allowance is available throughout the entire country, while the local authorities decide on the actual care services offered. In some municipalities, only the Caregiver Allowance is available, while in others both types of support can be offered simultaneously. This situation reveals the tensions within a policy subsystem with types of support within the same area regulated on a national or local level. A comparison of the number of beneficiaries of the Caregiver Allowance at 30 985 in 2005 and the recipients of care services at 4487, reveals the quantitative predominance of the allowance. In Estonia, the obligation of the family to take care of family members is defined by law, and the state is responsible only when the family is either not available or unable to manage care provision. However, men and women are gainfully employed almost to the same extent, with a low proportion of women working part time (European Commission, 2005).

According to official statistics of the Estonian Ministry of Social Affairs, in 2005 72.2 per cent of all informal carers were female (Estonian Ministry of Social Affairs, quoted in Kivisaar and Soots, 2006). A research project conducted by the Estonian Ministry of Social Affairs and the Estonian Association of Gerontology and Geriatrics confirmed spouses and children as the main informal carers, but also revealed an opening towards social networks composed of friends, neighbours and to some extent privately paid carers. The average age of the informal carers at 67 years is comparatively high. At 56.7 per cent, pensioners are quantitatively the most significant group, followed by domestic workers, that is, people staying at home (22.6 per cent). In contrast, only 10 per cent of the main informal carers are employed or self-employed (research results reported in Kivisaar and Soots, 2006). An explanation for the high proportion of domestic workers may be the decline of female labour market participation in the 55–64-year-old age group, and with a high proportion (78.5 per cent) of women among the carers within this age group (European Commission, 2005; Estonian Ministry of Social Affairs quoted in Kivisaar and Soots, 2006).

GOVERNING INFORMAL CARE THROUGH FUNDING: FUNDING PRINCIPLES AND SUPPORT STRATEGY

The analysis of governance of funding of informal care focuses on the mode of funding related to the different societal sectors involved (state, market, voluntary sector) and the level of funding. In all countries compared, cash payments are provided by the state or state-related actors such as social insurance on national or local levels, while the mode of funding (procedures and administration of the payments) and the level of funding differ. Levels and mode of funding are linked to the predominant support strategy selected in the compared countries, oriented either towards formal care provision or towards the provision of cash payments. Table 5.2 shows the relationship which is mapped out here, and the implications for carers demonstrated in the cross-country comparison. In addition to regulations, the mode and level of funding impact on the extent to which the boundary between formal and informal care has been shifted and informal care work has been formalised.

In Table 5.2, the different measures introduced in the countries selected are organised according to the level and mode of funding. Two levels of funding (more symbolically paid or oriented towards labour market wages) and two basic modes of funding can be discerned. Either the payments are directly paid to the informal carers or care receivers, or further agencies or organisations within the state, market or voluntary sector are involved. Moreover, a different pattern arises between countries oriented predominantly towards the support of informal care giving via care services and those oriented towards economic support of informal care.

Italy, Estonia and Germany, the countries preferring a transfer-oriented strategy linked to an emphasis on the role of the family, have introduced payments on a more symbolic level only which are paid directly to the informal carers or care receivers. In Italy, different allowances form the basis of public support within a transfer-oriented strategy. It is a fragmented system with different levels for application, eligibility criteria and so forth, and granted at either a national or local level (Lamura et al., 2001; Principi, 2005).[1]

Table 5.2 Predominant mode of funding

Economic support	To care receivers	To informal carer	Via state agencies	Via market	Via voluntary sector
Symbolic payment	*Germany* Cash benefits *Sweden* Attendance Allowance *Italy* Invalid Care Allowance	*UK* Invalid Care Allowance *Estonia* Caregiver Allowance	–	–	–
Related to labour market	*Sweden* Personal assistant (3%) *UK* Direct payments	–	*Sweden* Employed family carers *Sweden* Personal assistant (62%) *Netherlands* Care budget	*Sweden* Personal assistant (23%)	*Sweden* Personal assistant (12%)

On a national level, a state disability pension scheme has been established to provide an economic support after means testing to people with different types of disability. In addition, as a citizenship right on a national level a care allowance can be granted to 100 per cent disabled persons on the basis of certain defined criteria. It is a quite common allowance and about 6 per cent of the elderly aged 65 years and older receive this type of benefit (Polverini et al., 2004). Since the early 1990s, care allowances are increasingly granted by municipalities and regions as a supplement to the economic support provided at the national level and are generally means tested (Da Roit, 2005).

The situation reflects the paucity of formal care services together with the specific characteristics of the Italian 'cash for care' system. In contrast to formal care services, these care allowances and pensions are a statutory form of support that mainly falls under the remit of the national government implemented by the local authorities. While the national payments do not have any regional and local variations, at the local level considerable variations can be found, including even non-implementation, and the payments are often used to complement or even substitute for the provision of formal care services. They are principally used by beneficiaries and their families to hire migrant workers, who have become the most significant care pillar for many frail elderly. This has also been interpreted as a possible phenomenon of a new further stratification of the Italian society based on both gender and race dimensions. Labour market employment of many Italian women with frail relatives is possible due to the employment of female migrant care workers within their households or the households of their parents. Italian men only rarely take over caring responsibilities or caring tasks (see Andall, 2000; Colombo, 2003; Polverini and Lamura, 2004). Currently, migrant workers represent 83 per cent of all home care workers in Italy.

In Estonia, the emphasis on economic support of informal care provision can best be explained by developments comparable to the Italian case. As in Italy, in Estonia the family is legally responsible for care provision, formal care services have only limited availability, and the provision of cash payments as the dominant support strategy was unplanned. This situation is the result of task sharing between the national and local levels, related to the characteristics of the Estonian policy subsystem within the area. The Caregiver Allowance has been introduced on the national level, applicable throughout the country but with a sharing of responsibility between the national and local levels. While the local authorities are responsible for the application process and decisions, the national level was responsible for the funding until April 2005. The division of tasks accounts for the tremendous increase of beneficiaries between 2000 and 2005. The decision to grant Caregiver Allowances could lower the demand for care services provided and funded by the municipalities. Research on the application process in 2005 found that the local authorities granted 61 per cent of the applications for a Caregiver Allowance and 29 per cent of other allowances, including payments to buy care services. In 10 per cent of the cases the application was rejected and the family was assigned the responsibility for the care (Kivisaar and Soots, 2006).

The Caregiver Allowance is related to the level of care needs, but the payment is on a low level even compared to the wage levels in Estonia since the national allowance payment was €25.5 at most. Now the level of payment is decided by the municipalities and lies between €9.6 and €47.8, with up to €63.7 in exceptional cases. At the same time, the average income of a care receiver amounted to €180.9. The payment is made to a named care giver but there is no control over how the money is spent and it is expected to be complemented by payments of the care receivers and his or her family (ibid.).

In Germany, the emphasis on cash payments is not by default but is part of a strategy to support family care. The introduction of a cash benefit as one option within the framework of the LTCI was aimed at maintaining informal care within the family framework. Compared to the other available option, the provision of care service, the level of the benefits is needs related but the level of funding differs between both options. Cash benefits range between €205 and €665 per month and in-kind services between €384 to €1918 per month, making cash payments somewhat symbolic. Cost-containment strategies can partly explain the different levels of payment, but arguments related to the logic of the family have also been put forward. A payment for informal care work on the level of formal care provision, so the argument goes, also risks commodifying family relations. Furthermore, a more regular payment would demand a high level of control over the use of the money and the quality of the care delivered, which would be too difficult on a larger scale. In the course of the introduction of the LTCI, the disabled people's movement and the pensioners' organisations demanded the same level of benefits but were not successful (Meyer, 1996).

The benefits are paid to the care receivers and are mainly used to make symbolic payments to family members, neighbours and to some extent domestic workers, often with a migrant background, who are the so-called 'grey market' (Meyer, 2004). Despite the freedom of choice between cash benefits and care services, the socio-economic background is significant. Care receivers with lower socio-economic backgrounds more often vote for cash benefits. In contrast, the members of the upper middle classes more often choose care services (Blinkert and Klie, 1999). Klie and Blinkert (2002) revealed that people with a lower income more often opt for informal rather than formal care provision, due to economic reasons. In studies on the condition of informal carers, including an international comparison, a high level of exhaustion is evident in Germany which could be alleviated by the use of in-kind services (Giese and Wiegel, 2000; Schneekloth and Leven, 2003; Theobald, forthcoming).

In contrast to Italy, Estonia and Germany, where only symbolic cash benefits are available, in those countries that are oriented towards support via formal care services two types of benefits may be available. While symbolic cash benefits have been introduced earlier in some of the countries, more recently established policies differ considerably and have been developed within the framework of a more flexible care service provision, instead of the family framework with its goal of supporting family care linked to the logic of the family.

In both Sweden and the UK, care allowances related to more symbolic payments can be found but they differ with regard to their quantitative significance, the quality of social right and the influence of the local and national levels. In Sweden, under the Attendance Allowance established in the 1940s, there is no citizenship right but it is voluntary for the municipalities with local variations with regard to eligibility criteria and levels of funding. The decisions at the local level reflect the strongly decentralised policy subsystem related to the Swedish care regime with its high level of discretion for the municipalities based on the idea of local democracy (Rauch, 2005). The Attendance Allowance is paid directly to the care receivers and should be used to make a symbolic payment to a family member, friends or neighbours for help and assistance. In 2003, 7000 beneficiaries received a care allowance. The number of beneficiaries has decreased since the 1970s/80s with its peak of 21 000 Attendance Allowance recipients in the middle of the 1980s (Szebehely, 2005). The Attendance Allowance is mainly received by old-age pensioners, while women with a working-class and in particular with an immigrant background are over-represented. In many municipalities the allowance is the only type of support for the frail elderly with a migrant background (ibid.).

In the UK the Invalid Care Allowance was established in the 1970s and is a cash benefit that is paid to carers to provide a symbolic compensation for the loss of income due to caring activities. It is a part of the social insurance system and as such regulated through national legislation and available nationwide. The national government defines the eligibility criteria and the agencies of the Department of Work and Pensions administer the allowance. The local authorities do not play any role in relation to the allowance, thus providing an example of a centralised policy subsystem in the UK within the area of care for frail relatives. The allowance is a fixed and universal benefit in that it is paid independent of income and level of needs. The carers do not have to provide any evidence of the actual caring activities. In 2004, 425 455 persons received the Care Allowance, the majority being women (318 845 women as opposed to 106 610 men) (Department of Work and Pensions/ National Statistics, 2004).

In addition, in the service-oriented countries four measures have been introduced where the level of funding of informal care giving is related to labour market wages. The payments are not made directly to the informal carers or care receivers, and further societal sectors, chiefly the state or state agencies, are involved in the mode of funding. Both the higher level of cash payments and the more complex mode of funding related to a more intense control provide a starting-point for a formalisation of informal care provision. With the exception of the employed family carer in Sweden, the measures have been installed only recently. In Sweden the opportunity to be employed as a family carer emerged during the establishment of social care service for the elderly and can be explained as an example of the general trend to formalise informal care giving during this period (Szebehely, 2005). The carers are employed by the municipalities and, comparable to the Attendance Allowance within the framework of a strongly decentralised policy subsystem related to social care provision, the municipalities decide on the implementation of the programme and define further preconditions. This results in considerable local variations. The salary and the related social protections are comparable to those of the carer assistants in the local social services. The number of beneficiaries peaked in 1973 when 24 000 carers were employed though today only 3100 family carers are employed (ibid.). Employment as a carer is oriented towards informal carers of working age and is granted only in unusual situations such as where the care receiver lives in a very remote area (Johansson, 2004; Szebehely, 2005). Most of the carers are still gainfully employed, with only 10 per cent caring full time and 14 per cent retired. Like the Attendance Allowance, the benefit is used more often by women with a working-class or migrant background (ibid.).

The right to personal assistance in Sweden was introduced at a national level with the Law of Support and Service to Disabled People in 1994 for people with severe functional impairments. The regulations, in particular the eligibility criteria, are strictly defined by law (ibid.). The funding is provided by the municipalities for care needs at a lower level, but with increasing care needs the costs are granted by the national social insurance (Edebalk and Svensson, 2005). In contrast to the other types of cash payments for informal care giving, the national level provides a strict framework of regulations. The right to personal assistance is not meant primarily as a support strategy for informal care giving but rather as a strategy to provide a flexible care arrangement for severely functional impaired people. The beneficiaries are free to choose a personal assistant, who can be a relative or spouse. Approximately one-third of the beneficiaries living together chose the spouse or partner as a personal assistant. Moreover, there are different ways of organising such employment. The beneficiaries have the right to employ the personal assistant themselves, with the exception of the cohabiting partner or spouse, an opportunity which is only rarely used (about 3 per cent of the beneficiaries). The employment contracts are mainly administered by formal organisations, with a majority of 62 per cent of the personal assistants employed by the municipalities, a further 23 per cent employed by a private agency and 12 per cent by a user organisation. In 2003, 15 900 people in Sweden employed a personal assistant, with an average time granted of approximately 90 hours a week (Edebalk and Svensson, 2005; Szebehely, 2005).

In the Netherlands, the personal budget is available to beneficiaries approved by the national social insurance as one option besides in-kind services. The personal budget as the main cash benefit is based on the needs of the elderly person and funded in principle on the same level as in-kind services (Miltenburg, 2004). In 2001/02, the average care budget was €1308, corresponding to 65.5 hours per month. The number of beneficiaries has increased considerably over time, from 500 in 1996 to 70 000 in 2004 (Kremer, 2005). The personal budget is not directly given to the care receivers but is administered by the social insurance. According to recent changes, the calculation of the personal budget also takes into account the monetary contribution that the cared-for persons need to make themselves, which depends on the taxable income together with domestic circumstances. There are no distinct profiles among people opting for in-kind services or the personal budget (Miltenburg, 2004). According to Baarveld et al. (1998, as quoted in Tjadens and Duijnstee, 2000), a quarter of budget holders employ family carers and the overall majority of employed carers are informal carers. The carers outside the family framework are mainly women re-entering the labour market with an educational background in health care, and they work typically for one care receiver (Miltenburg, 2004).

In the UK since the 2002 Carers' Act, the municipalities have the right to introduce direct payments as an alternative to service provision. The national government strongly encourages the provision of this type of benefit as part of its policy of customer choice, although in practice the importance of direct payments remains limited. According to Lundsgaard (2004a), only 0.04 per cent of all people aged 65 years and older receive direct payments, with considerable local variations. The payments are given to the care recipients directly, but their use is very tightly controlled to ensure that the money is spent on the provision of care. In a qualitative study, Ungerson (2004) found that a number of care receivers employed only one carer, and a number of carers are working many hours for one care receiver only. She described how, despite the more-regulated situation, carers and care receivers are operating within a labour market with a low level of qualification and low wages and the carer is often working alone. There is a lack of support by agencies and both care recipients and carers have to find ways to organise the care themselves.

GOVERNING INFORMAL CARE THROUGH RULES: TOWARDS FORMALISATION OF INFORMAL CARE GIVING

The introduction of different types of cash payments allows regulating the – economically supported – informal care provision. The countries, however, differ widely as to whether and to what extent informal care giving has become an object of regulation. The newly established rules are imposed by the state, based on the state logic with its emphasis on hierarchy, laws and regulations. In addition, related to an employment contract, rules valid for the labour market may be involved. Three areas of informal care giving have become an object of regulations: the working situation or caring tasks of the informal carers; the quality of care provided; and the selection of the informal carers. In addition to the mode and level of funding, rules set up related to informal care provision define how and to what extent informal care has become a part of the formalised care provision. Table 5.3 provides an overview on the areas of regulations related to the different types of cash payments.

In Germany and Italy, two countries oriented towards a support strategy for informal care provision, the use of cash payments has been left almost unregulated. Decisions relating to the three defined areas are mainly made within the family framework, in other words the care recipient or his or her family decide on these issues based on their own needs or interests. This has created an overburdening care situation for informal carers related to the

Table 5.3 Rules related to cash payments

Areas	State	Labour market	Family framework
Working situation of the carer	*Estonia* Caregiver allowance	*Sweden* Employed carer Personal budget *UK* Direct payments *Netherlands* Care budget	*Germany* *Italy*
Care quality	*Germany* Cash benefits *Sweden* Personal assistant *Netherlands* Care budget *UK* Direct payments *Estonia* Caregiver allowance	–	*Italy*
Rules related to selection of providers	*Sweden* Employed carer Personal assistant *UK* Direct payments *Estonia* Caregiver allowance	–	*Germany* *Italy*

family logic with its emphasis on social or moral obligations as in Germany. It might also result in the employment of carers from a grey market outside the regulated formal care provision, as is often the case in Italy.

The one area of control is the weak but constant control of the care quality in Germany stipulated by the law based on the logic of the state. Professional care service providers specialised in these tasks control the quality of care provision on behalf of the LTCI. The frequency of the control visits is defined on a national level by law as twice a year in the case of a lower level of care dependency, and up to every three months in the case of the most frail. The objectives of the visits are to assess the quality of care and if it is not adequate to make suggestions as to how to improve the situation (Meyer, 2004).

In Estonia, the third country emphasising the economic support of informal care provision, in all three areas weak regulations and administrative procedures have been introduced that are related to the establishment of care provision (see Kivisaar and Soots, 2006). A care contract has to be signed by the informal carers and the local authorities, which defines the rights and obligations of both parties as well as payments. Both care receivers and informal carers have to agree to the contract. Within the contract, the working situation of the care giver is defined but the regulations and payments are not oriented towards formal employment. Moreover, the criteria for the selection of a care giver are very vague. Those selected can be neighbours, friends or family members but also individuals not acquainted with the care receiver, while gainfully employed family members are excluded. The care giver can be offered some type of training to increase the quality of care provision. After the allowance is granted there is no longer any quality control, that is, no control over whether the care giver actually provides the care or whether the provided care is appropriate to the care needs. Some cases of abuse have been reported, for instance, where the informal carer lives in another district, which raises questions as to whether the local authorities are following the regulations and administrative procedures. As a result, there are demands for additional regularised controls and support in daily care-giving activities.

In the countries oriented towards the support of home care via care services, different types of cash payments have been introduced. For comparison here, the measures with higher payment levels oriented towards labour market wages or more complex modes of funding are selected because they exhibit distinct differences with regard to the level of regulation. In Sweden, related to the programme of employed family carers by the municipalities, the criteria for the selection of carers are defined and the working situation is regulated according to labour laws with regard to wages and social protection. In most municipalities, this type of economic support is oriented towards family members of working age who reduce or have already reduced their working hours, but they are not obliged to end their employment on the labour market (see Johansson, 2004; Szebehely, 2005). The defined selection criteria with emphasis on family relatives reflects an orientation on the logic of the family based on kinship and moral or social obligation. The programme also integrates the logic of the state based on rules set up by the state and in particular even labour market regulations. Compared to the more symbolically paid informal carers, it provides a step forward to a more formalised regulated care provision.

The three measures only recently developed – direct payments in the UK, personal budgets in the Netherlands and personal assistance in Sweden – are targets of substantial control. These varied measures in three countries each allows the involvement of family members (restricted to family members outside the same flat or house in the UK), however, they are not oriented primarily towards family members but instead aim at enabling a more flexible care provision (Ungerson, 2003; Edebalk and Svensson, 2005).

In the UK, the carers have a formal employment contract with a payment subject to National Insurance contribution and they are typically paid for a specified number of hours (Ungerson, 2003; Lundsgaard, 2004a, b). However, there is a risk when friends or family members are involved of providing more support than is defined in the contract. This reveals the difficulties of combining a personal relationship based on the logic of moral or social obligations developed within social relations with paid work regulated by labour market laws. In addition, the level of regulation is defined by the labour market situation of carers in general. Ungerson (2004) points out that for the UK the level of regulation is low, reflecting the fact that the corresponding labour market is characterised by low wages, few skills and a lack of qualifications.

A further area of regulation concerns caring activities. In the UK, the expenditure on care activities has to be documented through a paper trail linked to a very tight control that shows that the money provided is spent on care provision and not used to pay a family member living in the same accommodation. Payment presupposes a full documentation of the caring activities and evidence that the care worker pays National Insurance contributions. In the Netherlands, the care recipients receive only a small amount of the granted money. Instead the money is mainly administered by the social insurance office and is paid upon receipt of documentation of the caring activities and evidence that the contracts with the carers meet legal obligations (Miltenburg, 2004). In Sweden, when the beneficiaries act as an employer, they are responsible for documenting the caring activities for the insurance and fulfilling their obligations as an employer. The overwhelming majority (97 per cent) do not act as an employer – rather, the municipalities, the private agencies or user groups take over the responsibility, including the documentation and the employer obligations. They are obliged to provide a thorough documentation, oriented towards the caring situation as such. In an amendment of the law, the municipalities, private agencies or voluntary organisations are obliged to aim for a good quality of care provision and proper adaptation to the individual situation of the users (SOS, 2005b).

In general, due to the orientation towards informal carers, even outside the family framework the employment contracts corresponding to wages and regulations on the labour market and the control of the caring activities provide a starting-point for a more formalised care provision. However, the mix of logics (of the state, the (labour) market and the family), the weak employment situation of carers on the labour market as such, and the limited orientation towards a control of care quality impede the formalisation and, if used on a larger scale, may even be a risk for the development of a secure labour market position for carers and an adequate care provision.

CASE STUDIES

The cross-country comparison of the integration of informal care provision revealed two basically different modes: either more family oriented or more service oriented. The Netherlands and Italy are selected as case studies in order to analyse the process in greater detail. In the Netherlands, the idea of state responsibility for the provision of care services has been well established since the end of the 1960s. The introduction of personal budgets that include informal care can be seen as part of a strategy to develop further care provision within a corporatist care system that traditionally involved state and non-state actors, but increasingly also representatives of carers' or users' organisations. In contrast, in Italy the idea of family responsibility has resulted in an uncoordinated approach to supporting family care economically, enabling families to find solutions for care needs privately. Only recently have efforts been made on the national level to develop a more coordinated approach, by including different state and non-state actors such as unions and the employer organisations and different carers' or users' organisations.

Personal Budgets and Voluntary Care in the Netherlands

Karel de Bakker and Trudie Knijn, University of Utrecht, the Netherlands

Home care governance in the Netherlands is designed to provide care for patients requiring long-term specialised care that is not covered by standard health insurance policies. The scope of this care is broad in the types of care that it provides. This is reflected even in the name of the 'Algemene Wet Bijzondere Ziektekosten' (AWBZ) law or 'universal law for specialised health care costs', in place since 1968. The original purpose of the law was to ensure care for those people who were chronically ill, handicapped, or needed to be taken into care homes. Over the years, however, more aspects of care were incorporated (in particular, home care) and with the personal budget (PB) a new type of benefit that includes informal care provision has been established.

The integration of voluntary care: personal budget

The AWBZ employs two mechanisms for delivering care to people.[2] Care can be delivered either by recognised care organisations or users can decide to receive a PB, that is, financial help meant to provide them with the means to find their own care giver privately. The amount provided for the PB is determined by calculating the care needed based on intensity of care and hours required (anything from cleaning help to professional nursing care) and then subtracting from that their own personal amount (calculated for all recipients for both in-kind services and PB based on their household income).

One of the more interesting aspects of the PB is that it enables the care recipients to compensate financially volunteer care givers who are known personally to the care recipient, including relatives, for their caring activities. The ability to pay volunteer care givers for their help means that the recipients are able to choose the type of care they prefer and give financial support to the care giver, while providing long-term intensive care that may take them away from work. While this is a good way to provide care to those who need it without tying up health care institutions, it is important to note that according to the AWBZ, certain care such as nursing must be provided by a qualified professional.

The question of paying those who provide voluntary care was recently raised as an issue that may require extra attention, specifically as to whether paying voluntary care givers would monetarise voluntary care. The conclusions reached by studies carried out by the CVZ (College Van Zorg Verzekeringen, an independent organisation that studies and mediates in matters of public health care) and the ITS Nijmegen (Nijmegen research institute) were that the use of the PB to pay voluntary care givers did not result in a significant change in attitude among the care givers. Between 65 and 75 per cent[3] of paid care givers interviewed would have been providing help whether they were being paid for it or not. In addition to this, the study showed that a voluntary care worker who was paid with a PB worked on average 8 paid hours a week and a further 14 unpaid hours a week. It was decided that the advantages of allowing people with a PB to hire people they knew as care givers outweighed any fears of the monetarising of voluntary home care. Indeed, it was also felt that care workers deserved to receive more support for the work that they do.

As of the start of 2006, there were almost 80 000 people in the Netherlands who received a PB under the AWBZ and it is believed that this number will continue to grow.[4] The expansion of the PB system is attractive to the users as it gives them control over their own care as well as providing support to the voluntary care workers who often sacrifice aspects of their own lives to care for others. In addition, the PB system means reduced cost to the government (typically voluntary carers provide more care than they are paid for and the costs for administration are reduced) and a step towards the government's goal of reintroducing the idea of members of the community caring for one another.

The changing face of home care: devolution of responsibility to the local level

The current mood in home care governance is that of providing personal care to the recipients at a more local level. In relation to this, 2007 will see the introduction of a new law known as the *wet maatschappelijke ondersteuning* (WMO; community support legislation) in which many of the smaller care functions which previously fell under the AWBZ will be taken over by local governments. In addition, other legal statutes dealing with specialised health care will be bundled together to be regulated by local government, such as laws pertaining specifically to the handicapped as well as social support for those with long-term medical problems. Care recipients will be able to find all the information they need in one place as a result of the WMO taking several care laws under its wing and it should be more efficient in ensuring that all recipients receive the care to which they are entitled. In fact, one of the stated objectives of the change is to reinforce the idea of community or social support by making it easier from a governance standpoint for members of communities to care for one another by making the system more accessible and limiting bureaucracy to a single regional office (Landelijke Vereniging van Indicatie Organen, 2003). Not without reason, commentators fear that more obligations will be imposed on (female) family members by stricter definitions of care needs. Indeed, the national guidelines for 'usual care', introduced in 2003, include strict criteria that members of the household have to fulfil themselves before any additional care will be provided by the AWBZ. Within a year, the AWBZ reduced the number of definitions of care needs by 30 per cent (Centrum Indicatiestelling Zorg, nd).

By 2007, home care in the Netherlands will be split, in a sense, into three spheres:

1. AWBZ, which will apply to those in need of specialised care such as care homes, medical treatment and admission to medical facilities.
2. WMO, which will apply to those who require more personal aid in and around the home such as cleaning, help with caring for children, social interaction and other care often provided by voluntary care givers.
3. PB, which will give care recipients the ability and freedom to decide for

themselves what kind of care they receive and when by providing financial compensation. PB is possible within the framework of both the AWBZ and the WMO systems.

Issues in home care and actors involved

The main issue for debate in political forums concerning home care has been government-controlled or free market home care organisations in the Netherlands. In the early 1990s, Dutch parties from the political left such as the PvdA (Partij van de arbeid/social democrats) and the SP (Socialistische partij) argued that privatisation of home care would lead to higher costs, lower quality and a more financially driven rather than quality driven home care system for the customer. At the same time, parties such as the VVD (right-wing liberal) and the CDA (Christian democrats) argued that free market competition would be beneficial to home care. Competition over patients would mean that costs would be lower and quality would need to be retained if home care providers hoped to retain their client base (Verhagen, 2005). By the late 1990s, a compromise was eventually reached which would see private and public home care organisations sharing the market. The overall response to this was quite positive as most people felt that the quality of the service they had received was at a high level.

While the political discussions surrounding home care are one part of the debate, the corporatist model of decision making in the Netherlands means that every decision made concerning possible policy changes in home care is influenced not only by political parties but also by unions and other representative organisations, who each get a say in forming the policy that will eventually affect them. For example, the above-mentioned CVZ was asked by the government to put together a report pertaining to the significance of certain issues that were to be subject to change. In addition to organisations representing the care providers there are others, such as Per Saldo, which with 16000 members represents the interests of people who receive a PB.[5] During a government debate a few years ago concerning a newly published report which recommended that PBs should not be spent on volunteers, Per Saldo reacted negatively, and the government asked the CVZ to produce a report examining the issue. Through such negotiations everyone receives representation and a compromise is reached that should lead to an effective solution.

Home care in the Netherlands is growing rapidly; an ageing population means that the issues and actors involved in the governance of home care will become more important in the future, as will the ability to provide quality care to not just the elderly but also to the chronically ill or those suffering from long-term injuries. Realising the growing importance of home care, government, industry and care recipients' representatives use a dialogue in the corporatist tradition to reach effective solutions to problems. The expansion of the PB and allowing care recipients to pay voluntary care workers for the time and effort they put into caring for their friends and loved ones is an example of how this functions. All this means that discussion and compromise in home care governance will aim to make home care in the Netherlands accessible, flexible and of high quality, where all actors have their say and where people are compensated for the work they put in while caring for others.

Italy's 'Familistic' Approach to Elderly Care and the New Role of Migrant Home Care Workers

Giovanni Lamura, Italian National Research Centre on Ageing, Ancona, Italy

The peculiarity of Italy's welfare system in the European and international context of elderly care has traditionally been characterised by a family-based approach, combined in the most recent decades with a substantial transfer of public resources to families in the form of care allowances aimed at enabling them to 'perpetuate' their caring role. More recently this approach has facilitated an increasing employment of migrant home care workers who have de facto become one of the fundamental pillars of the current Italian LTC 'system'. A system in 'inverted commas' since this situation has never represented an explicit aim of Italy's official elderly care policies but rather a pragmatic solution adopted by families to face the demographic and socio-economic changes.

Demographic and socio-economic changes: unmet needs

This evolution of the Italian way of caring is the result of the combined effect of several actors and processes that can be outlined as follows. From a *demographic* point of view, a growing care demand is the natural consequence of Italy's position as the country with the highest percentage of the population aged 65 years and over (Kinsella and Phillips, 2005: 7). This situation is reflected by a rapidly worsening *potential support ratio* (that is, the ratio between the number of adults aged 15–64 and the number of older people aged 65 and over (United Nations, 1999: 48)) which is eroding the quantitative reserve of adults available to take care of dependent older people. More relevant is the reduction of the availability of informal care deriving from *socio-economic trends*, such as the increasing female participation in the labour market (the female activity rate almost doubled between 1972 and 1994 to 42 per cent, increasing to 51 per cent in 2004 (OECD, 2005a:16)) and the reduction of support from social networks available to older persons (reflected by a reduction in the number of multigenerational families and an increase in the number of elderly living alone, but also by the reduction in the number of older households receiving external informal help (Sabbadini, 2003)). However, these changes have not significantly affected the 'familistic' thinking of most Italians, who continue to be among the least convinced in Europe about the state's responsibility for elderly care. Over 80 per cent of them consider it a 'good thing' if in the future 'working adults would have to look after their elderly parents more than nowadays' (Alber and Köhler, 2004: 65 and 78).

The peculiar role played by informal care in Italy and its recent changes cannot be thoroughly understood, however, without considering the parallel evolution that recently occurred in the formal care sector. It is worthwhile remembering that according to Italian law, any person requiring care can count on the following support sources: free health care from the national health system; means-tested social care from municipalities (whose amount, however, depends on available funds); care allowances from both the state – in terms of (means-tested) disability pensions and (non-means-tested) care payments of totally dependent persons – and a growing number of local authorities (that is, regions or municipalities, generally means tested); alimony (that is, economic support to cover living costs, including those deriving from increasing care needs) from relatives up to the second degree, which is an individual right granted by law (Lamura et al., 2001). All these forms of support have undergone major changes in the last few years and the combined effect has pushed Italian families to search for a 'private' solution to their growing and changing care needs. Efforts to rationalise the hospital system have caused a sharp decrease in the average length of hospital stay (Ministero della Salute, 2004). This in turn has contributed to an increase in the number of inappropriate admissions of dependent elderly to old people's homes, for which some regions have introduced user co-payments in the case of longer stays (Tinti, 2004). Financial constraints and lack of appropriate planning have prevented regions and municipalities from introducing a more systematic enlargement of formal home care services, despite the preference given to this form of support by Italian families (Alber and Köhler, 2004: 72). Thus local authorities have increasingly opted for integrating already existing state care allowances with further own-care payments (Pavolini, 2004: 207–8; Da Roit, 2005: 198–9) in order to support families in the choice of continuing to care for older people at home, or preventing or delaying the much more costly institutionalisation for the municipalities.

Informal care and migrant carers

The introduction of different types of monetary transfer has produced a situation where a totally dependent person can benefit from between €1000 and €1250 per month from different – and not always integrated – public sources. These have been increasingly used by families to privately hire migrant home care workers, often on a live-in basis (Gori, 2002; Polverini and Lamura, 2004). A major reason for the development of this trend lies in the wage differentials existing between Italy and the migrants' sending countries, increasingly from Eastern Europe after the first waves from the Philippines and Latin America (Lamura et al., 2006). Furthermore, to keep costs low this often occurs on an undeclared basis by hiring illegal or legal immigrants without a legal contract. In order to deal with this phenomenon, in 2002 the Berlusconi government legalised '*una tantum*' the position of over 340 000 illegal home care workers and introduced yearly 'immigration flows' specifically addressing this category of migrants, among others. In 2006, over 45 000 of them benefited from this quota system, and by the end of that year the Prodi government was already debating the possibility of legalising a further 100 000 migrants who applied over and above the available places.

On the whole, this process has produced both a strong expansion of the available home care workforce and its transformation into a real ethnic niche. Over the last 15 years, the number of home care workers (including housekeepers) has increased from 180 000 in 1991 to about 700 000 in 2005. The number of foreign nationals increased from 16 to 86 per cent! Migrant care workers have therefore de facto become a fundamental pillar of the Italian LTC system, for several reasons: their economic convenience (the cost of a co-resident care worker to the hiring family is about half that for residential care, and is now also fiscally deductible); the tailored care they provide (caregiving families appreciate in particular the care continuity and timeliness they ensure, preventing dramatic changes in their own lifestyle, including the harmonisation of work and care); the delay or complete prevention of institutionalisation (between 1991 and 2001, a further decrease of 40 to 50 per cent in the already relatively low use of residential care occurred among the over 85-year-old population, see Tomassini et al., 2004); and the economic advantages for migrant workers themselves due to the high income differentials. However, the widespread employment of migrant care workers in Italy raises questions of quality of care in terms of the need to improve the qualifications and training of often totally unprepared migrant care workers (Lamura et al., 2004), integration with existing formal care services, functioning of the labour market and exploitation of migrant care workers.

Steps to a more coordinated policy development

In the light of this complex situation, the Prodi Italian government is now trying to revise current policies for the provision of long-term care by providing a more systematic and integrated approach between formal and informal care providers based on the following key points (Ministero dell'Economia, 2006: 140–41): the creation of a national LTC fund, incorporating the different sources currently available under different budgets; strengthening of integrated home care services; definition of nationwide 'essential care levels'; and adoption of a national bill on home care workers in order to bring to light undeclared care work and define common requirements to improve their professional skills and reliability as well as grant higher care continuity to users and their families. Whether these aims will actually be realised will largely depend on how Prodi's government will be able to achieve a concerted action with the other relevant social parties.

The trade unions in principle welcome the re-proposal of the LTC fund (the first proposal was blocked by the right-wing government at the end of the 1990s, officially for lack of funding). On the other hand, trade unions are afraid that the costs of such a fund might be borne by cutting public expenditure in other relevant areas. Indeed 'pensions' and other 'health care services' have been mentioned by the current Prodi government as possible candidates for such cuts. Employers' organisations have commented less on the proposal regarding the LTC fund and are much more concerned about the need to reduce labour costs for their enterprises. A much more relevant role is played in this respect by other volunteer and non-governmental organisations involved in the care sector, such as the Alzheimer Federation and Association, disabled people's organisations, and volunteer organisations providing care and support to dependent older people, all of which have strongly pushed for the introduction of the LTC fund in previous years and now hope that the new Prodi government will finally be able to take the right steps in allowing the LTC fund to become a reality: a major challenge that will soon reveal to what extent Italian society is able to properly take care of its weakest members.

NOTES

1. We should like to thank Dr Giovanni Lamura, National Research Centre on Ageing, Ancona Italy for his information on the situation in Italy.
2. See www.pgb.cvz.nl/.
3. See Uitvoeringsverslag PGB Nieuwe Stijl (2005).
4. Ibid.
5. See Per Saldo.

6. Care workers: defining the boundaries of occupational territories

As the previous chapters illustrate, home care is high on the political agenda across many countries and in many instances this leads to various processes of formalising care arrangements. Various new funding schemes in formal care services are an example, as are the introduction of payments for informal carers. In relation to care workers, processes of formalisation, especially as they occur under tight financial constraints, raise issues about the boundaries between care workers with different levels of training on the one hand and boundaries between paid care workers and informal carers on the other (see Ewijk et al., 2002; Boom et al., 2004). Such issues often point to underlying conflicts between professional and economic rationales and lead to the redefinition of boundaries in terms of different processes of reskilling and deskilling. This chapter examines these processes across countries against the background of underlying governing arrangements that make for varying degrees of institutionalisation of care work as an occupational activity, and that in turn are related to broader contextual factors of the governance of home care.

The following analysis focuses on paid care workers who deliver formal care services as part of formal employment and who tend to have formal training or even formal qualifications. It uses a typology developed by the European Foundation for the Improvement of Living and Working Conditions (2006), which includes traditional formal carers working in the public sector or the private for- and non-profit sector, independent formal carers registered with employment agencies and personal assistant carers personally recruited and employed by individual care recipients and/or their families. As the discussion of informal care in Chapter 5 demonstrated, however, the boundary between the formal and the informal is blurred and traditional formal carers work side by side with personal assistant carers. Moreover, traditional formal carers at the assistant level often have as little formal training as personal assistant carers. The analysis here requires going beyond identifying boundaries and mapping out the dynamics of and conflicts over a set of boundaries within the context of redefining boundaries in terms of processes of reskilling and deskilling. In this respect, it is also important to note that the statistics available on the workforce in home care are very patchy (Moss and Cameron,

2002). For example, for Italy, New Zealand and the US only estimates are available and relevant international datasets are incomplete. This makes it very difficult to use figures as a basis for cross-country comparison, and thus in the following analysis we use figures only in an indicative way.

As suggested above, the logic of the family is a salient element of the governance of care workers because the family continues to be the primary location of care work. Yet as Chapter 3 on the contexts of home care governance demonstrates, there are interesting variations of this logic that can be expected to impact on the governance of care workers. For example, as illustrated in the analysis of formal care services in Chapter 4, a gender culture that is based on the primacy of formal care in the context of female full-time employment as typical of the dual breadwinner/institutional care model offers favourable conditions for the development of formal care services. The conditions are less favourable in a gender culture that puts family care first and sees women as part-time employees or housewives. Because care workers are the main providers of such services, this also has implications for the governance of care workers. The relative level of support for formal care services provides more or less favourable conditions for care workers to be a comparatively well-defined area of governance. In the context of his analysis of nursing across six European countries, Dent (2003), for example, points out how the relative importance attached to familialism and subsidiarity impacts on the relative institutional standing of care work as an occupational activity. This reflects differences as to whether the state considers women as wives/mothers or workers and to what extent the state protects against the market. Benoit and Heitlinger (1998) and Theobald (2003) present a similar argument in their respective comparative analyses of women's care work and elderly care.

CARE WORKERS AS PROVIDERS: VARIANTS OF WEAK INSTITUTIONALISATION

In relation to care workers as providers, the relative institutionalisation of care work as an occupational activity is related to the level of qualification, ranging from unqualified but possibly trained care assistants to care workers with specialist qualifications in non-hospital-based care. It is also related to the relative differentiation of the occupational structure. Both are important indicators of the prevalent balance between formal and informal care in individual countries. In this respect the relative focus on formal care services provides more or less favourable conditions (see Kerkstra and Hutten, 1996; Escobedo et al., 2002). This reflects the fact that the existence of formal care services is often an indication of the settledness of funding arrangements and this provides the material basis for a labour market for care work. At the same time, the level of qualification in itself may not always be a precise indicator of the relative institutionalisation of care work as an occupational activity. For example, an extensive provision of formal care services may mean the inclusion of basic care tasks that require only low levels of training. Both the relative level of qualifications and the relative differentiation of the occupational structure are also closely related to where formal home care services are located in relation to the divide between health and social care services, as well as how formal care services fit into the overall organisation of welfare. The occupational orientation of care workers may be more or less strongly oriented towards health and social care, respectively. The former are often characterised by higher levels of qualification and a more differentiated occupational structure than the latter, thus reflecting the firmer institutionalisation of health care in the welfare state. Table 6.1 offers an overview of our countries.

As suggested earlier, home care cuts across the boundary between health and social care and, as Chapter 4 demonstrated, countries have taken different approaches to defining that boundary and to organising health and social care-based home care services. This also influences the relative balance between care workers with a health care/nursing-based occupational orientation on the one hand and a social care-based occupational orientation on the other. In Germany and New Zealand, care workers with nursing-based qualifications/training are the largest group among the workforce in home care whereas in the UK, Estonia and the Netherlands, care workers with social care-based qualifications/training dominate. Sweden by contrast is a case of a hybrid orientation. Japan is difficult to characterise, as formal care workers are a very recent phenomenon. Finally, Italy and the US pose interesting cases where personal assistant carers with extremely weak occupational orientations dominate.

The UK is a typical example of a country where social care orientations are dominant among care workers in home care and where this closely corresponds to the specific divide between health and social care services. Historically, care of the elderly in their own home has had a marginal position compared to other welfare services, reflecting its transitional nature (Malin, 2000). This type of care is concerned neither with cure (as is the case with health care) nor with the moral integration of society (as is the case with mental health care). At the same time social care has been marginal, not only in relation to health care as the main national welfare service but also in relation to other (mainstream) welfare services provided by local authorities such as education (Means et al., 2003). In turn, the peripheral and unspecified organisational position of social care has made it difficult for a distinct occupational structure to emerge.

This contrasts with health care where a grading structure makes for a highly differentiated occupational structure that also includes specialist (community) nurses. As such, care workers in (social) home care are also particularly strongly exposed to and affected by organisational reforms, and here the introduction of market reforms since the late 1980s is an indicative example. The reforms challenged care workers from below with the emphasis on care *by* the community and from above with the emphasis on management. The more explicit inclusion of informal care as part of the notion of a *mixed economy of care* challenged the position of formal (and by extension qualified) care, and as such potentially makes for the deskilling of care workers (Malin, 2000). Managerialism for its part had more ambivalent effects. On the one hand, qualified care workers moved into management, pointing to a process of reskilling, and this meant a de facto deskilling of the delivery of care itself (Cameron and Moss, 2001). The training of front-line carers also has a primarily in-house character and focuses on ensuring the functioning of services as opposed to the development of professional practice. However, with the parallel shift from health to social care services the occupational scope of (social) care workers has de facto become broader and included more health care activities (Cameron and Moss, 2002a).

In the case of Sweden, care assistants are the predominant group of care workers and their occupational training programme of care assistants includes both social and health care components. Training provides the basis for employment in the delivery of either health or social care, making for a hybrid occupational orientation. The training is also a prerequisite to studying nursing care or social care at a university of applied sciences (SOS, 2003) and it is only at this more advanced level that the two orientations are more clearly distinguished. In contrast, for care assistants the setting they work in is decisive for the principal type of service they deliver. This is further strengthened by the fact that many care workers acquire their vocational training on the job. The hybrid occupational orientation of care assistants is also reflected in developments at the level of service organisation. Traditionally, social care services were provided by the municipalities oriented towards a social model, while home nursing organised by the county councils was oriented towards a medical model. Since the 1990s, however, the increasing cooperation between social care services and home nursing care, together with the targeting of services towards more frail care recipients, has strengthened the medical orientation of social care provision (Trydegard, 2003). Therefore even in relation to social care the care assistants deliver the daily caring activities, while nurses organise and supervise the care provision. In summary, the scope of skills of care assistants as the largest group of care workers is clearly limited and closely related to the specific requirements of the workplace.

Table 6.1 Overview of characteristics of care workers delivering formal home care services

Country	Characteristics
UK	Majority have social care orientation, only minority have health care orientation *Health care* • differentiated occupational structure with different levels of nursing including specialist community nurses *Social care* • predominance of home helps with minimal training • 80% of staff do not have relevant qualification, but focus of work is increasingly health-care related
Estonia	Great majority have social care orientation, only a very small minority have health care orientation *Health care* • predominantly registered nurses (graduate nurses or nurses with vocational training between 2 and 5 years) • many staff work part time *Social care* • 70% of staff have (two years) vocational training/further training as social care worker
Germany	*Health/social care* • majority of staff (40.3%) have nursing-based orientation and among those, fully-qualified nurses dominate • second-largest group (28%) have further/no training • third-largest group (17.8%) have social care-based qualification
Italy	Overwhelming majority are personal assistant carers (est. 88.2%) with extremely weak occupational orientation, formal carers represent a very small minority *Health care* • flat occupational structure with registered nurses only • recently recognition of 'support role' of 'social-health workers', who deliver care under supervision of medical/nursing staff *Social care* • 2-tier occupational structure with social workers (3-year university-based training) and home helps (basic education)

Japan	*Health/social care* • many staff are registered and practical nurses • growing proportion are certified welfare specialists • minority are untrained or have minimal training with pressures to import more carers from outside
Netherlands	*Health/social care* • differentiated occupational structure in both nursing and home help, but only minority (7.7%) are nurses, over half of staff are care workers (51.2%) • majority (40.6%) have medium- (as opposed to high-) level qualification; 15.9% have low-level qualifications
New Zealand	*Health/social care* • about 50% (est.) of staff have a health care orientation, but of those about 80% at assistant level • about 10–20% (est.) of staff in social care have social work qualification (diploma or 3-year university degree); the remaining staff have limited or no formal training or qualification
Sweden	*Health/social care* • great majority (75%) have hybrid health/social care orientation at assistant level; among those only about half have 2–3 years training
US	Majority of staff (64.3% est.) are personal assistant carers with extremely weak occupational orientation; formal carers represent a minority of staff *Health care* • predominantly registered nurses • minority are licensed practical nurses or nurse aides with limited training *Social care* • minority formally trained in social work in associate degree (2-year) programmes

Sources: Hutten (1996); Kerkstra (1996); Japan Ministry of Health, Labour and Welfare (1999, 2002); US Department of Health and Human Services (2000, 2001, 2004); Cameron and Moss (2001, 2002a, b); Davey (2002); Ewijk (2002); Ewijk et al. (2002); SOS (2003); Polverini and Lamura (2004); Theobald (2004); New Zealand Federation of Voluntary Welfare Organisations (2005); Kivisaar and Soots (2006); Personal Comunication Giovanni Lamura, National Research Centre on Ageing, Italy.

Together with the US, Italy is an example of a country where personal assistant carers with an extremely weak occupational orientation make up the largest group in the home care workforce. The care workers are mainly declared or undeclared migrants, many of whom have a high level of education and are trying to use care employment as a stepping stone for other types of employment (Hillmann, 2005). Specific agencies are increasingly involved in the recruitment of such migrant care workers (Socci et al., 2003) although the employment itself is controlled by individual care recipients and/or their families. Employment conditions are therefore highly variable, and depend on the specific household at hand. Nevertheless, in many cases employment is permanent yet causal, and based on a live-in arrangement. Polverini and Lamura (2004) describe the central role played by migrant personal assistant carers as the major change in the provision of home care in Italy. What are the explanations of this change? A first explanation relates to the paucity of publicly funded services and associated shortages of formal care workers (Socci et al., 2003). Underlying this is a general lack of public support of the family that reflects the longstanding struggle between the opposing views of the Christian Democrats and the Communists (Polverini and Lamura, 2004). This lack of public support has become especially problematic against the background of the more visible limits of family capacity related to increasing female labour market participation (Socci et al., 2003; Hillmann, 2005). Finally, the existence of highly unregulated cash benefits offers ample incentives for the employment of personal assistant carers.

The discussion of the relative health and social care occupational orientation of care workers suggests that social care orientations dominate, and that this is also closely associated with a relatively weak institutionalisation of care work as an occupational activity. The often weaker position of social care in welfare states means that care workers with a social care orientation tend to be characterised by a less differentiated occupational structure together with lower levels of training/qualification, compared to their counterparts in health care. At the same time, some countries such as the UK have also seen an explicit move away from health to social care. Altogether this means that overall, the relative institutionalisation of home care work as an occupational activity is low although there are clear differences at the extreme ends of the continuum. The variations among countries point to interesting, country-specific combinations of different aspects of the institutional context of home care governance, especially the relative support for female employment and for formal care services, respectively.

The US and to an even greater extent Italy are examples of countries where the overall level of qualification of care workers is very low, indeed where the majority of care workers are personal care assistants, many with a migrant background. This illustrates the fact that there is a considerable need for paid workers in home care, reflecting the conflicting demands that the dual breadwinner/part-time female carer model puts on women in terms of being both part-time carers and full-time employees, while the means-tested care regime clearly limits the public support for formal care services. The majority of home care workers are either employees of private home care agencies or hired directly by clients or their families. Although in recent years the Medicaid programme has placed increasing emphasis on home care, it remains largely a residential-centred programme. Moreover, since Medicaid is heavily means tested and generally serves only the most indigent, most elderly persons do not qualify. As a result, often the most qualified and registered workers tend to work in institutional centres while the home care workforce has disproportionately been drawn from a less-qualified and less formally trained pool, including a much higher proportion of minorities, foreign nationals and immigrants who are generally paid low wages with few benefits, including health care. As a result, turnover of home care workers in the US is higher even than for other carer groups.

In the Netherlands, and the UK in relation to health care, there exists a relatively differentiated structure of relevant qualifications, while the overall level of qualifications is also low. A possible explanation is that the public service model as encapsulated by the Social Insurance for Exceptional Medical Risks was historically closely associated with elderly care in institutions. In contrast, a familial orientation has been stronger in relation to home care. Also Knijn (1998, 2000) suggests that the post-war history of home care has been a continuous effort by government to control funding through regulating the pay and working conditions of care workers. Historically, home helps emerged as casual supporters of mothers who were temporarily unable to cope. It was only later that formal qualifications came to be considered, but this focus had already begun to fade in the 1970s. Budget cuts provided the basis for the first moves towards deskilling, which took the form of recruiting unskilled part-time workers. These were typically married women who were looking for part-time jobs. The introduction of the so-called 'alpha helps' who were to be employed through the existing provider organisations formalised this form of employment. Beyond economic considerations this also reflected a support for the status of housewives on the part of the government. This made for a weak occupational field, which the introduction of market mechanisms since the late 1980s further challenged.

The personal care budget is an example of the new and potentially conflicting demands from users as consumers in four respects: the status of professional knowledge, professional authority, professional orientations towards the public good, and the trust between professions and their clients (Kremer and Tonkens, 2006). More specifically, there are no a priori qualification requirements and users have a genuine choice between formal and informal carers and potentially also between formal carers from different provider organisations. Formal care workers (typically home helps) are therefore under a certain pressure to show that they are worth their money. The highly individual employment settings also mean that home helps may be confronted with demands that go beyond their skills or even against professional standards (Kremer, 2005). Home helps also have little scope for developing their professional knowledge and education (Kremer and Tonkens, 2006).

In contrast, the overall level of qualifications among the workforce in home care is higher, although to varying degrees, in Estonia, Germany and Sweden. In the case of Sweden, this resonates with a care regime where formal care services are available universally and that is underpinned by ideas about the preference for formal over informal care and for female full-time employment. In conjunction with the fact that the majority of care workers are women, the latter expresses a commitment to the formalisation of women's work and as such also provides a springboard for the governance of care workers. In the case of Estonia, the higher levels of qualification point to the tensions between a care regime where state support for formal care services and female labour market participation is low, and one where women's employment is high and mostly full time. Together with the challenges of managing the aftermath of the economic and political transition from communism, this has provided a catalyst for improving the educational level or training of care workers and nurses (Kivisaar and Soots, 2006). In 1999 a two-year vocational training programme for social carers was introduced, and in 2000 the former vocational training of nurses was re-established as part of higher education and the period of education increased to 3.5 years. In addition, further training is offered to social care workers and nurses already employed in areas with low overall levels of training. Finally, the case of Germany highlights two specific aspects of the organisation of care services: first, the predominance of health care service where the focus has been on securing mid-range levels of qualifications and second, the stark separation between informal and formal care, which resonates at the level of ideas with a preference for family care.

In summary, the analysis suggests two things. Besides differences at the extremes, the governance of care workers as providers is characterised by a continuum of relatively low levels of qualification that often correspond with an occupational orientation on social care and a weak differentiation of the occupational structure. The variations point to a number of factors, including the relative emphasis on formal care services (for example, Sweden and Italy) as well as country-specific constellations of sometimes conflicting ideas and different aspects of care regimes.

PAYING CARE WORKERS: COMPLEX VARIATIONS OF COLLECTIVE AND INDIVIDUAL AGREEMENTS

In relation to care workers, funding is concerned with issues of paying them. Paying care workers includes issues surrounding the regulation of salaries (and working conditions) where countries vary concerning the relative importance of collective as opposed to individual agreements. Variations across countries are in part related to the characteristics of care workers as providers in terms of levels of qualification and specialisation as well as the characteristics of work settings, including health care versus social care settings and public versus private settings. Variations across countries also reflect the type of industrial relations predominant in individual countries. Table 6.2 provides an overview of our countries.

Table 6.2 suggests that there is considerable variation in relation to the existence of collective agreements (mostly at the national level) and individual agreements at the level of individual employers (or even with individual employees). In Sweden, the Netherlands, Italy and Japan as well as in Germany (in relation to employees of public/private non-profit providers) and Estonia (in relation to nurses) collective agreements exist whereas in the UK, the US, New Zealand, Germany (in relation to private employers) and Estonia (in relation to social workers) individual agreements dominate. In part the regulation of salaries and the relative importance of collective agreements are related to the specific organisation of labour relations in a country (Bamber et al., 2004). In the US, for instance, in many areas of the country home care workers are classified as 'independent contractors' who under federal anti-trust laws are banned from unionising or bargaining collectively (Schneider, 2003). This reflects highly liberal labour relations together with the liberal welfare state regime typical of the US. One of the main reasons for employing home care workers as independent contractors is so that employers do not have to pay for health insurance.

Even in countries where collective agreements are a key element of labour relations, however, the regulation of salaries of care workers can be fragile, illustrating the often weak institutionalisation of care work as an occupational activity and the low status of care workers as compared to other occupational fields in welfare. In Japan, for example, the otherwise highly regulated corporatist model of labour relations is much less well defined in relation to care workers. Reasons for this are that care workers represent a rather recent category of workers and are not very strong in numbers. Collective agreements and salary negotiations of public home care workers take place at the provincial level. Although traditionally Japanese home care workers were employed by a mix of public and non-profit voluntary organisations, under deregulation there has been a large increase in for-profit suppliers (more than

Table 6.2 Regulation of salaries of care workers

Country	Collective vs. individual agreements
UK	Mainly individual agreements at local level
Estonia	*Nurses*: collective agreements at national level *Social care workers*: individual agreements at local level
Italy	Collective agreements applied to all care workers; different agreements in the public and private sectors
Japan	Collective agreements; agreements at local (municipal) level but within national guidelines
Germany	Collective agreements with private non-profit providers; mainly individual agreements with private for-profit providers; collective agreements with welfare associations at national/local levels depending on individual association
New Zealand	Individual agreements; agreements at district level, although in principle national; government has capacity to regulate (but as yet has not done so)
Netherlands	Collective agreements
Sweden	Collective agreements; agreements follow national framework but include local adaptations; within that framework negotiation of individual wages supplements
US	Individual agreements; much variation by locality and no national policy; unionisation of care workers increasing across states

Sources: Hutten (1996); Kerkstra (1996); Cameron and Moss (2001, 2002a, b); US Department of Health and Human Services (2001); Ewijk (2002); Ewijk et al. (2002); Fujiwara et al. (2003); Schneider (2003); SOS (2003); Davey and Keeling (2004); Karlsson et al. (2004); Polverini and Lamura (2004); Theobald (2004); Kitchener et al. (2005); Noguchi and Shimizutani (2005); Kivisaar and Soots (2006); Personal Comunication Giovanni Lamura, National Research Centre on Ageing, Italy.

22 000 such institutions in 2000) which is fragmenting the collective bargaining base (Noguchi and Shimizutani, 2005). There are also explicit moves to open the corporatist system of labour relations to facilitate the employment of migrant care workers.

The regulation of salaries of care workers also often depends on the specific organisational settings they work in. Are they employed in the public or the private sector and do they work in a health care or a social care setting? Labour relations are often more firmly established in the public sector and in relation to health care settings, thus providing a favourable basis for collective agreements. As such, any moves of the provision of formal care services from the public to the private sector and from health care to social care settings potentially have considerable implications for the regulation of salaries of care workers.

In the case of Germany, for example, the opening up of formal care services to private providers as part of the introduction of the long-term care insurance (LTCI) has undermined the predominance of collective agreements and now individual agreements prevail. Before, service providers associated with the major welfare associations primarily stood for the delivery of home nursing care. The welfare associations established their own collective agreements that were modelled upon the collective agreement in the public sector. In contrast, for private for-profit care providers, individual agreements prevail and wages differ significantly from those paid under the collective agreements in the public sector. Also the wages of managerial staff are often considerably higher than those of staff involved in daily caring activities. The recent collective agreements of the welfare associations have tried to follow the developments in the for-profit sector. The competition among providers within the emerging care market together with strict cost containment policies further pushes developments in this direction (Theobald, 2004).

New Zealand for its part is an example of the other dichotomy, where the regulation of salaries varies between health and social care settings. Only health care workers have collective agreements under district health boards. Despite the recent integration of health and social services, such agreements do not apply to most other home care workers. This reflects the fact that care workers in health care are public employees and well organised, while the social care end of home care is newer and as such weakly institutionalised. The Nurses' Organisation, Service Workers' Union and Fair Share Campaign are among the forces now calling for a well-trained workforce with collective protections.

In summary, the governance of care workers through regulating salaries is characterised by the existence and sometimes co-existence of both collective and individual agreements. At the same time, moves towards strengthening private providers and the expansion of the provision of social care-oriented services often coincide with moves towards individual agreements. Variations across countries point to a complex mix of different factors, including the relative institutionalisation of care workers as providers (for example, the contrast between home nurses and home helps in New Zealand) and broader patterns of labour market relations (as experienced in the US).

RULES IN RELATION TO CARE WORKERS: HIERARCHY AND CONTRACTUALISATION

In substantive terms, rules in relation to care workers are concerned with the regulation of (minimum) levels of qualification required for care delivery and the regulation of the occupational territory of home care workers. They are interesting as they involve studying hybrid forms of rules (for example, Knijn and Verhagen, 2003; Verhagen, 2005; Knijn, 2006). As discussed above, the logic of the family is salient and the regulation of home care workers has traditionally been marginal to the governance of the welfare state. Instead, association and market-based rules, especially by providers collectively or individually as the employers of care workers, have been more important.

The relative balance among different types of rules is changing, however. The formalisation of care discussed in Chapter 4 regarding the governance of formal care services, including the formalisation of informal care, gives primacy to hierarchy, while the deskilling of certain lower segments of the care workforce is likely to be associated with market and association-based rules (especially in the form of contracts). The importance of the logic of the state resonates with analyses of feminist research in the sociology of professions that point to the central role of the state in occupational projects of female care workers (see Witz, 1990; Wrede et al., 2001; Henriksson et al., 2006). However, studies often show that the more extensive the role of the state in welfare the more strongly institutionalised the position of care workers. Benoit and Heitlinger (1998), for example, contrast the minimal patriarchal welfare state in Canada and its very limited support for paid health care work with the institutional partnership welfare state in Sweden with its extensive women-friendly employment policy. Theobald (2003) observes similar differences in the relative professionalisation of care of the elderly in her comparative study of Sweden and Germany. The same applies to Burau's (2005) study of community nursing in the UK and Germany. Table 6.3 presents an overview of our countries on this measure.

Across our countries, hierarchy plays a central role in the regulation of the qualifications of care workers, including minimum requirements in terms of qualifications and training. At the same time, the importance of hierarchy in relation to the levels of training can be deceptive as the de facto scope of such regulation may be limited, thus reflecting the overall low levels of qualification. For example, Japanese care workers are a relatively new phenomenon, and levels of qualification are low. The same holds for New Zealand despite the integration of social care with health care, where the level of qualification remains considerably higher. An even more extreme case is Italy, where the regulation applies only to a very small minority of care workers since the majority are personal assistant carers.

Rules based on hierarchy are often relatively new. In Japan, for instance, the regulation of qualifications of care workers has traditionally been disjointed. Under the LTCI, attempts have been made to standardise qualification and training. In the 2005 reform, measures were implemented to strengthen the required teaching credentials and curriculum in the care worker certification programme. A revised national examination has been put in place to encourage a standardised curriculum at training facilities across prefectures and secure national educational consistency. Likewise, the newly established National Training Qualification for care workers in New Zealand is an attempt to encourage a standard certification process that will link pay levels with qualifications.

The hierarchical regulation of work-based qualifications of care workers therefore is relatively extensive, particularly where it concerns the lower segments of the occupational structure. Such regulations may be an indication of relatively extensive governing resources, although in the case of the UK this occurs as a hybrid with association-based employer regulation. The expansion of market mechanisms since the late 1980s has had an ambivalent impact on the governance of care workers. The mixed economy of care has led to a marked increase in the number of private providers and thereby further fragmented the already weak career structure in social care (Cameron and Moss, 2001). The impact of contractualism has been similar and has been an impetus to break up established patterns not least because it coincided with a strong emphasis on cost efficiency (Malin, 2000). This trend points in the direction of market-based regulation through micro-level decisions by employers.

At the same time, however, the government has increasingly defined the framework of such decisions. Regulation occurs first and foremost through managing local authorities and the regulation of the private market, but this has provided a springboard for extending the focus of control from services to work itself. In this respect, the introduction of national vocational qualifications is indicative (Thornley, 2003; Johansson and Moss, 2004). Within this scheme, employers as members of sector-specific skills councils define national occupational standards, and as such the standards are principally work related and competence based. This scheme helps by integrating existing skills to a national standard, yet the skills are narrowly focused to fit a specific task,

Table 6.3 *Regulation of the qualifications and occupational territory of care workers*

	Regulation of levels of training[1]	Regulation of occupational territory[2]
Hierarchy Regulation through legal/ quasi-legal provisions	*UK* Through national vocational qualification definition of skills and recognition of training of health/social care staff without formal qualifications *Estonia* National level regulations define curricula for nurses and social care workers *Germany* Federal law defines content of vocational training *Italy* In the case of nurses and social workers through national educational system; in the case of home helps and social-health workers through regional vocational systems *Japan* National examination regulates qualification of care workers; recently revised to help standardise curriculum across different training facilities *New Zealand* District health boards (as public funding organisations) together with professional and provider organisations (including Primary Health Care Nurses' Council, NZ Federation of Voluntary Welfare Organisations, and Access Homecare) define training/qualifications required	*UK* Indirectly, through national-level regulation of training of health/social care staff without formal qualification; indirectly, through national guidance on implementation and inspectorates defining and controlling standards of service in health and social care *Estonia* Indirectly, through national-level regulations of curricula for nurses and social care workers *Germany* Indirectly, through federal law that defines content of vocational training; directly, through federal social insurance legislation: within specialised nursing care some tasks can be conducted by (fully qualified) nurses only, within basic nursing care (fully-qualified) nurses retain overall responsibility but may delegate tasks to other staff *Italy* Indirectly, through national laws defining content of educational curricula for nurses and social workers, and regional laws defining the training contents for home helpers and social-health workers; directly, through national legislation identifying which tasks are nursing care, social care and 'basic'

	Sweden National legislation defines the content of nursing (university) education (that leads to subsequent registration); same applies to the vocational training of social carer/nurse assistant, but which is not a formal prerequisite for employment	care (by home helps and social/health assistants) *Japan* Directly through national LTCI guidelines to municipalities; indirectly, through the national examination that regulates qualification of care workers and national fee structure that regulates formal care services *New Zealand* Indirectly, through definition of training/qualification requirements by public funding organisations and professional/provider organisations *Sweden* Indirectly through national legislation that defines contents of nursing education (that leads to subsequent registration) and social care (although the latter not very important in practice); directly, through binding regulation by the National Board of Welfare that defines that nurse in charge may delegate tasks to individual staff members
Associations Regulation through professional self-regulatory bodies, provider organisations or trade unions	*UK* Professional self-regulatory bodies define (and monitor) qualifications of qualified nurses and social workers *Netherlands* Trade unions and professional organisations together with employer organisations and organisations representing vocational colleges decide on the required skills and corresponding qualifications of care workers	*UK* Indirectly, through professional self-regulatory bodies defining qualifications of qualified nurses and social workers *Netherlands* Indirectly, through social partners defining qualification for care workers; indirectly, through contracts between providers and insurance funds defining the scope of formal care services in context of social insurance

Table 6.3 continued

	Regulation of levels of training[1]	Regulation of occupational territory[2]
		US Directly through Medicare/Medicaid guidelines and waivers to states for publicly funded care workers only; indirectly, at state level and through national carers' associations; care service unions and private care service companies
Market Regulation through micro-level economic decision	*Italy* As part of (un)declared employment of personal assistant carers individual care receivers and/or their families decide on the required competencies/training *Sweden* Service providers (mainly municipalities) decide if individual carer is employed as nurse assistant or at lower level *US* Market driven though some state governments have introduced minimal requirements for registered care givers	*Estonia* Directly, through micro-level decisions by local providers (mainly municipalities); home nursing requires nursing qualification at either graduate or vocational level; in social care staff conduct the same tasks irrespective of level of vocational training *Italy* Directly, through micro-level decisions by individual care receivers and/or their families as part of (un)declared employment of personal assistant carers

Notes

1. This refers to any regulation of (minimum) levels of training required for care workers to provide formal home care services and includes the level at which regulation occurs.
2. This refers to any regulation of what formal home care services encompass and includes the level at which regulation occurs.

Sources: Hutten (1996); Kerkstra (1996); SOSFS (1997a, b); SOS (1999); Malin (2000); Cameron and Moss (2001, 2002a, b); US Department of Health and Human Services (2001, 2004); Davey (2002); Ewijk (2002); Ewijk et al. (2002); Japan Ministry of Health, Labour and Welfare (2002); Fujiwara et al. (2003); Schneider (2003); Thornley (2003); Davey and Keeling (2004); Karlsson et al. (2004); Polverini and Lamura (2004); Theobald (2004); Kitchener et al. (2005); New Zealand Federation of Voluntary Welfare Organisations (2005); Noguchi and Shimizutani (2005); Kivisaar and Soots (2006); Personal Comunication Giovanni Lamura, National Research Centre on Ageing, Italy.

thus pointing to the tensions inherent in an initiative where government supports employment-based training (Malin, 2000).

Compared to hierarchy, other forms of rules are less important. For example, professional self-regulation as a form of association-based rules exists in few countries and almost predominantly in relation to nurses, who in most countries represent only a small group among care workers. Nurses are also the group of care workers whose position is particularly well institutionalised in the (health) division of labour. In the UK, for instance, an independent statutory body, the Nursing and Midwifery Council, maintains a register for qualified nurses, sets standards of conduct, performance and ethics, and monitors such standards through dealing with cases of malpractice.

The explicit market-based regulation of qualifications is equally rare and among our countries existing only in the US. Despite a growing presence of the federal government in home care under Medicare/Medicaid, regulation continues to be largely market based in the US. This is reflected in the prevalence of casual employment by employment agencies that mostly hire staff as independent contractors and of casual employment by individual care recipients and/or their families. Nevertheless, the Home Health Quality Initiative (2003) supposedly will rectify the lack of federal oversight by closely monitoring home health quality measures, although its coverage does not extend to other care workers. In 2001, over 2.5 million elderly persons received care from over 7000 Medicare certified home health care agencies. Moreover, over 15 per cent of the elderly were covered by private long-term care insurance in 2001 and this is growing rapidly. Public regulation such as exists in some states tends to focus on entry requirements only.

By contrast, in other countries such as Estonia and Sweden, elements of market-based regulation exist within an overall hierarchical approach to regulating the qualification of care workers. This also demonstrates the close relationship between state and market-based forms of regulating qualifications, and by extension the occupational territory of care workers. In Sweden this hybrid form of regulation is closely related to the distinction between nurses, and health and social care assistants. Employment as a nurse requires an examination in nursing at university level together with a registration with the National Board of Health and Welfare. Despite the existence of a national vocational training programme for social care, no such requirements exist in relation to the employment of care workers or care assistants. Instead, employers themselves can define the criteria to be used to assign an employee to the occupational group of health or social care assistants (SOS, 1999). This is of critical importance in an area of care provision where most of the employees acquire their vocational training as part of their job based on the specific opportunities offered by employers.

The relatively strong embeddedness in and even dependence on the state means that care workers are also particularly vulnerable to reforms of the welfare state, and reforms have often played a central role in the redefinition of the occupational boundaries of care work, by default rather than design (see Knijn and Verhagen, 2003; Henriksson et al., 2006). An important recent example is the introduction of market mechanisms in welfare. In relation to home care this has taken a number of forms, including the introduction of contracts that is often accompanied by the emergence of private providers. Compared to other countries, the introduction of market mechanisms in home care has come a long way in the Netherlands (Knijn, 1998). The introduction of managed competition in the late 1980s followed far-reaching budget cuts and associated mergers of care providers, starting in the 1970s. The central idea was to use profit making as a means to stimulating competition among providers so that providers would deliver quality care at the lowest possible price. More specific measures included allowing private, for-profit providers into the delivery of formal care services; tailoring services through complex processes of needs assessment; facilitating the integration of social and health care services; and introducing personal budgets to strengthen user choice. The measures were not only numerous but also reflected competing logics (Knijn, 2000). For example, while service providers are meant to compete with each other they are also expected to cooperate with each other to strengthen the integration of service provision. Similarly, while personal budgets are supposed to allow for user choice, the use of funds is subject to tight bureaucratic regulation. These tensions have led to an extreme fragmentation of the system of home care (ibid.).

Although these developments do not in themselves change the regulation of qualifications as such, they have further and potentially considerable implications for the *scope* of such regulations. Contractualisation, with its focus on putting a price on explicitly defined services, challenges the professional logic (which in our typology is a variant of the logic of associations) and thus puts considerable pressure on care workers with formal qualifications and training (Knijn, 2006). Here the pressure is twofold, and includes both a push towards employing less qualified and trained care workers and one towards formalising informal care work through the introduction of different forms of payment (discussed in more detail in Chapter 7 on the governance of care users). Germany and the Netherlands are prime examples of this and are discussed in more detail as part of the case studies below.

As such, the contractualisation of care work also has considerable implications for the regulation of the occupational territory of care workers in home care. These pressures have tended to be indirect, and regulation has occurred mainly through education in that the curricula content gives an indication of what care workers are able to do. More explicit regulation of occupational territory through contracts has been typical of countries like Germany, the Netherlands and Japan (in relation to those aspects of home care that fall under the health care insurance) where the funding of formal care services is based on social insurance. In Japan, the uniform fee schedule has largely been effective in setting allocation priorities and thus also regulating health care occupations. It serves as an allocation mechanism by providing a financial incentive structure for the provision of selected services (that is, primary care) by setting the fee allowed higher than the actual costs. In contrast, because no extra billing is permitted, the fee structure can discourage medical applications deemed undesirable by setting the allowable fees lower than the actual costs. The fee schedule is not only a 'powerful tool' for promoting certain services and thus shaping the distribution of health care resources (Ikegami, 1992: 691) but also exerts considerable influence over the practice of health care occupations.

In some cases this even includes the explicit definition of what differently qualified staff are allowed to do. In Germany, for example, the regulations differ with regard to specialised or basic nursing care. Specialised nursing care is carried out on the basis of a referral of a medical doctor and funded only within the framework of the health care insurance. As part of a medical treatment, specialised nursing care includes activities such as giving medication and controlling blood sugar. The activities have to be conducted mainly by trained nurses. In contrast, within the LTCI framework, only basic nursing care (for example, support or assistance with activities of daily life such as washing, eating and mobility) are provided. Management and coordination activities are reserved for trained caring staff, that is, nurses or elderly carers, while nursing and elderly care assistants respectively may deliver daily caring activities under the guidance of trained staff. Supported by regular visits from trained staff, even informal family carers are allowed to provide basic nursing care (see case study below).

The new contractualism builds on these developments and represents a considerable extension of explicit regulation (Knijn, 2006). Here conflicting trends of exclusion/deskilling of some care workers and inclusion or reskilling of others (informal, specialists) are connected to market-based regulation by default, in the sense that a considerable part of the care workforce is not qualified. Considering the high plasticity of care work, care workers therefore have substantial problems maintaining their professional status together with their occupational uniqueness.

In summary, the regulation of the rules of the qualifications and occupational territory of care workers based on the logic of the state dominate, but in some countries they are combined with rules based on association and the market. Such hybrid forms of rules have gained ground with the increasing contractualisation typical of recent market-oriented public sector reforms. As a result, the regulation of occupational territory in particular has become more explicit. The variations among countries are numerous but often highly specific and it is therefore difficult to systematically point to underlying contextual factors.

DISCUSSION AND CASE STUDIES

The analysis of governing arrangements as they relate to care workers offers a number of insights into the governance of home care more broadly. Our countries are characterised by an array of variations in terms of the relative institutionalisation of care work as an occupational activity. The relative differentiation of the occupational structure together with the relative level of qualification characterises care workers as providers (with the extremes of the predominance of personal care assistants and a relatively well qualified workforce within an overall low level of institutionalisation). Moreover, the relative strength of collective agreements is central for care workers as employees with complex variations across countries. Finally, the relative importance of different types of rules characterises the regulation of care workers where hierarchy prevails, increasingly in the form of hybrids with rules based on profit seeking.

The variations across our countries reflect a range of contextual factors, including the relative emphasis on formal care services, country-specific constellations of ideas and aspects of care regimes, and specific features of the organisation of formal care services. Together they offer more or less favourable conditions for the occupational development of care workers as trained and paid employees. In conclusion, this is an area of governance that illustrates the centrality of the private and the associated logic of the family relative to an area of governance that is very much related to the public sphere. It also highlights the centrality of state in the regulation of paid care work largely irrespective of variations in relation to contextual factors.

Against this background the remainder of the chapter presents two case studies, one from the Netherlands and the other from Germany. Despite differences in their respective governing arrangements and the underlying contexts of home care governance, the care workforce in both countries is subject to processes of reskilling and deskilling. As such, the two cases offer an opportunity to examine in more detail the interplay between ideas and institutions together with the dynamics among actors. In the Netherlands, market-oriented public sector reforms have provided a platform for new hybrid forms of state and market-based governance and, together with salient tensions underpinning the context of home care governance, have led to the partial reskilling and considerable deskilling of the care workforce. In

Germany, by contrast, the governance is now more strongly based on the logic of the state. This state of affairs reflects the introduction of the LTCI and, in conjunction with specific salient features of the organisation of formal care services, has led to the partial reskilling and some deskilling of the care workforce.

Dutch Care Workers in the Context of Hybrid Forms of State and Market-based Governance[1]

The Netherlands is an interesting case for understanding the dynamics of the governance of care workers and associated processes of deskilling and reskilling. The institutionalisation of care work as an occupational activity is relatively strong, the occupational structure is differentiated, collective agreements are the norm, and hierarchical regulation of care workers has existed for some time. This epitomises a care regime that is built on the public service model and where the provision of formal care services has long been well established. At the same time, the Netherlands is also a country where market-oriented public sector reforms have been particularly strong. The reforms have mainly been concerned with the organisation of the delivery of formal care services together with the integration of informal care, but they have also had wide-ranging effects on care workers and have challenged the institutionalisation of care work as an occupational activity from both above and below (see Knijn, 2000; Boom, forthcoming). This section examines the central ideas underpinning the reforms and the views of key actors and discusses individual aspects of the reforms and the effects they have had on both the governance of care workers and on care work as an occupational activity. It argues that present processes, especially of deskilling, reflect not only recent hybrid forms of governance but also salient tensions in the institutional context of the governance of home care.

The market and the cost-efficient use of resources have been the predominant ideas underlying wide-ranging reforms of health and social care services since the late 1980s. In relation to home care more specifically, four ideas are particularly relevant (see Knijn 1998, 2000): integrating home nursing and home help services to avoid unnecessary overlaps and to provide services tailored to needs; a mixed economy of welfare with both non-profit and for-profit private providers to stimulate competition; detailed assessment of care needs by external agencies to ensure tailored and cost-efficient service delivery; and strengthening the influence of users through the introduction of personal budgets. These ideas are related mainly to the organisation of care delivery, but they point to other underlying ideas about care workers. In terms of care work as an occupational activity, the ideas are mixed (also see Boom, forthcoming) and include the idea of care work as a generic occupational activity, that combines both nursing and home help tasks; the idea of needs assessment as a bureaucratic activity that is separate from the occupational activity of service delivery; and the idea of informal care work as a formal care activity. In terms of the governance of care workers, the underlying idea seems to be one of a hybrid form of governance that combines strong elements of state-based governance through the detailed definition of care needs and assessment procedures with some elements of market-based governance, especially through micro-level decisions by care users but also through competition among providers.

The Netherlands is characterised by a corporatist consensus-oriented approach to policy making that includes different societal actors. In relation to the reforms of home care, the policy process has been characterised by an emerging consensus between government and societal actors but one which crucially has not included professional interests. In his analysis of the public debate from the 1990s onwards, Verhagen (2005) suggests that until 1997 the views of government and social actors were characterised by major differences about the balance between the public and the private, especially in relation to the delivery of services. In contrast, developments since 2000 have been characterised by a more pragmatic approach, with government and social actors looking to balance the market with continued state involvement. In comparison, the views of professionals have been less influential and the conflict between the professional and the economic logic has remained intact. Professional groups continue to criticise the focus on form rather than content, which they see as undermining the motivation of care workers.

What is the substance of the reforms and what are the implications for care work as an occupational activity and the governance of care workers? The integration of home nursing and home help services has not only increased the size of providers but has also put the division of labour between the two types of care workers into the spotlight (Boom, forthcoming). The latter has occurred especially in conjunction with a process of detailed needs assessment. In conjunction with the focus on cost efficiency and containment, this has led to a clearer differentiation between highly skilled care management on the one hand and less skilled front-line delivery of care on the other. Furthermore, the assessment of care needs and the principal allocation of care tasks are now in the hands of independent statutory assessment agencies at the regional level. The agencies define care needs and associated care activities following detailed provisions that form part of the regulation of the Social Insurance for Exceptional Medical Risks. This points not only to the partial deskilling of care management (ibid.) but also to the strengthening of rules based on hierarchy at the expense of rules based on professionalism as a variant of the logic of associations, in this case in the form of micro-level decisions by front-line professionals. A similar process but from the opposite direction has occurred with the introduction and gradual expansion of care budgets (on the broader context of this debate, see Knijn and Verhagen, 2003). The potential availability of informal care is now also part of the process of needs assessment, and thereby informal care emerges as a care activity on a par with formal care. The training and payment of informal carers point towards a similar direction and mark the increasing formalisation of informal care as an occupational activity (Kremer and Tonkens, 2006; Boom, forthcoming). In addition, care users also become employers of care workers (especially home helps) and thereby the 'custodians of professional development' (Kremer, 2005). In terms of the governance of care workers, the care budgets introduce rules based on competition (in the present case in the form of micro-level decisions by care users) as well as in conjunction with the needs assessments and the administration of care budgets strengthens rules based on hierarchy (ibid.).

In summary, the strengthening and partial redefinition of state-based governance and its combination with elements of market-based governance has in part weakened the institutionalisation of care as an occupational activity (Knijn, 2000; Kremer, 2005; Boom, forthcoming). This analysis emphasises the importance of conjunctional factors in the form of market-oriented public sector reform, together with the interplay between government and major societal actors. However, the weakening of the institutionalisation of care work as an occupational activity did not come out of the blue but instead is connected to salient tensions in the institutional context of home care. As discussed earlier in this chapter, historically the emergence of the public service model is closely related to the development of institutionally-based care services, and has been less strong in relation to home-based care services. Here it is indicative, for example, that in relation to home helps the focus on qualification and training has been less strong since the 1970s and instead low-qualified alpha helps have become the main group of care workers (Knijn, 2000). This coincides with the fact that there is also a large pool of women potentially available for this type of work. Compared to other countries, female labour market participation is low and mostly part time thus reflecting limited state support for female employment together with ideas about subsidiarity (see Knijn, 2001; Boom, forthcoming).

Reskilling and Deskilling Home Nursing within the Long-Term Care Insurance in Germany

With the introduction of the LTCI in Germany in 1995/96, long-term care was accepted as a social risk which has to be regulated and funded on the basis of an independent social insurance. The definition of long-term care as an independent area together with new regulations of responsibilities and working tasks within the area were not at first intended to change the status of nursing care, but in effect resulted in processes of deskilling and reskilling of nursing activities. The establishment of long-term care as an independent area led to a decisive push for the professionalisation of nursing care in general. In contrast to the regulations of the statutory health care insurance where only the medical doctors have the right to diagnose an illness and to decide on appropriate treatment, within the framework of the LTCI, nurses have the right to assess independently the level of care dependency. In addition, as the lead service providers it is mainly nurses who develop the provision of care services and who negotiate fees with the insurance funds. The definition of a distinct and independent occupational area for nurses and the creation of some independence *vis-à-vis* the dominating medical profession was a novelty in the German health care system (see Landenberger, 1994). The medical doctor associations, which were not very interested in the issue of long-term care in general, criticised the development and suggested (unsuccessfully) the involvement of family doctors in the process of needs assessment (Meyer, 1996).

While there is general agreement that the definition of a distinct occupational area has strengthened the position of nurses towards the medical doctors, the effects of LTCI on the professionalisation of nursing care within daily care provision is much more ambivalent. According to the law, long-term care has to be provided under the guidance of a nurse or elderly carer in charge and other carers such as nursing assistants and volunteers. Furthermore, within the family framework informal carers may conduct the necessary care activities supported by regular visits from nurses. It was envisaged that within home care provision, qualified nursing staff would be active mainly in key areas like management and coordination of formal care provision and counselling, while the basic caring and housekeeping activities should be delivered by nursing assistants, volunteers and informal family carers.

The reaction of the nurses and their professional associations to these legal provisions was twofold. On the one hand they saw the risk of deskilling: the increasing involvement of nursing assistants in formal care provision and the recognition of informal family care may lead to a declining status of care activities. On the other, the definition of a management role for nurses coordinating the work of nursing assistants and counselling informal family carers were judged as an opportunity for a further professionalisation of nursing care (Welti, 1999a). The strategies of professional associations were extended to include the issue of cooperation between qualified nursing staff and other paid and informal carers. In a report for the Deutscher Verband für Pflegeberufe, one of the two main professional associations, the designation of management, coordination and evaluation as activities to be conducted by trained nurses or elderly carers only was suggested as a professionalisation strategy. The emphasis on the cooperation with other carers in the law, however, prevented a more comprehensive strategy (Igl and Welti, 1999; Welti, 1999a, b).

The five non-profit welfare associations as the main care providers held the opposite view (see Meyer, 1996). They supported the recognition of informal family care and the involvement of voluntary workers as a traditional element of their care provision. Furthermore, from their perspective not all caring activities have to be conducted by qualified caring staff. In contrast, since the 1980s the welfare associations have demanded financial resources for the employment of more qualified staff during cost negotiations with insurance funds or state authorities. In the course of the development of the LTCI law, the welfare associations successfully argued for making high-quality standards a goal of care provision. This was to counterbalance the focus on price and definitions of quality by the insurance funds, which were seen to be motivated mainly by the aim of cost containment.

The demand for care provision following evidence-based standards resulted in new legislative provisions but also provided the starting-point for further professionalisation efforts by nurses, their professional associations, and scientific societies associated with nursing schools (Landenberger, 1994). They unsuccessfully demanded an independent organisation for quality assurance. Since the introduction of the LTCI, however, two laws have come into effect to improve the quality of daily care provision. First, a new federal law for the training of elderly carers, the Training Staff in Elderly Care Act, helped to standardise the different vocational training programmes on a relatively high state level. Second, the Quality Assurance and Consumer Protection Act required providers to introduce quality assurance measures into the insurance funds to assess and monitor the quality of care services.

According to the law, high-quality standards in care provision should be achieved without raising insurance contributions, and these conflicting objectives have impacted on care workers in a number of ways. The umbrella organisations of service providers have employed nurses with university degrees to develop quality assurance programmes. However, this comprises only 0.28 per cent of the staff within formal home care provision (Federal Statistical Office, 2005c). In addition, about 6.36 per cent of the caring staff, mainly nurses with vocational training, are involved in management or coordination activities (ibid.). Despite its low status, the increased demand for formal carers in basic nursing care has been met by employing for the most part qualified labour (Gerste and Rehbein, 1998; Federal Statistical Office, 2005c). Instead, an increase in part-time work and more flexible working-time patterns are the main strategies to lower costs. At the same time, private for-profit providers have increased the wages of management staff and have lowered the wages of front-line care workers (Theobald, 2004).

The comparably high level of qualification in home care also reflects the fact that qualified care staff are more flexible and can deliver services under both social insurance schemes (Federal Statistical Office, 2003). Moreover, even the LTCI largely covers basic nursing care, whereas the share of housekeeping tasks is small (Federal Statistical Office, 2005b). Despite an expansion of formal care provision, informal family carers continue to deliver most of the care. In 2003, 68.5 per cent of the care receivers living at home opted for cash benefits only, and organised their care provision mainly within the family framework (Federal Statistical Office, 2005c). The quantitative significance of informal family care giving contrasts with the generally qualified caring staff within formal care provision, and reflects a sharp boundary between formal and informal care. The high proportion of informal care delivery forms the basis for the stable insurance contributions.

NOTE

1. The literature available in English is limited and we are therefore particularly grateful to Hannerieke van der Boom (University of Maastricht) for allowing us to use her chapter on the Netherlands, which is part of a forthcoming cross-country comparative study on home nursing (Boom, forthcoming).

7. Care users: between citizens and consumers[1]

Changing conceptions of the role of the users in social care provision mark a key element of home care reform in most Western societies. Several debates have contributed to the newly defined role of the users in care provision (see Ungerson, 2003; Clarke et al., 2005; Clarke, nd). Debates on processes of individualisation in society question whether existing forms of care provision are responsive to the increasing diversity of needs and wants among the care users. Social and user movements have been raising their voice against dominance and dependency as a characteristic of the traditional relationship between care users (clients) and the professionals in public service provision. Social or citizenship rights related to care are emphasised as a way to expand the traditional male-oriented model of citizenship. Social rights, empowerment, autonomy of the users and freedom of choice within service delivery are catchphrases reflecting the debates.

The demands put forward within the debate can be related to competing approaches to care delivery with their emphasis on different logics of governance (see Chapter 2 and Knijn and Verhagen, 2003; Vabo, 2004; Clarke et al., 2005). Laws and regulations introduced and imposed via hierarchy as a part of the logic of governance by the state are emphasised as a starting-point for the establishment of social rights, which aim at supporting an equal treatment of the users on the basis of democratically controlled bureaucratic administrative principles. Here the empowerment of the users on the basis of social rights is viewed as a precondition for a more individualised care delivery. In contrast, consumerist ideals related to the market logic of governance view the user choice between service providers as a prerequisite for a more individualised care provision. On the basis of competition between different types of care providers in a care market and the introduction of freedom of choice for the users, a more individualised care delivery should be possible. The family-oriented approach characterised by the logic of kinship is based on values such as moral and personal obligations and reciprocity. The recognition of informal family care is viewed as a basis to secure care provision in general. Additionally, the freedom of choice between formal and informal care delivery is emphasised as an opportunity for care adapted to individual needs.

The newly introduced care policies for a more individualised care provision combine efforts to introduce or redefine social rights and regulations linked to the state logic of governance, efforts to enhance freedom of choice for the users as characteristic for the market logic of governance, and efforts to include family care giving based on the family logic of governance. The interplay of the state and market logic of governance within the new care policies is at the centre of the chapter (for a discussion of the family logic, see Chapter 5, on integrating informal care). Despite common assumptions, the redefined conceptions of the users and their relationship to social service reform and the measures introduced differ among Western countries. In the following cross-country analysis, the changing conceptions of users and their embeddedness in public debates and social care reforms in general as well as the measures introduced and their consequences for care provision are discussed. This section proceeds on the assumption that the new mix between state and market logic and the introduced social rights are influenced by:

1. the policy subsystems in the countries, in particular the interplay of the local and national levels which define the impact of the introduced changes on the entire country;
2. the orientation of the care regimes towards the market and the state, which generates a general openness or resistance towards the introduction of market principles; and
3. the quality of social rights related to the care regimes as the precondition for the use of different types of user choice.

This discussion contributes to the understanding of home care governance in several ways. First, related to the logic of the market, the establishment of a care market with competing public, private for-profit/non-profit providers aims at facilitating user choice among different options. In our countries, a tension arises between the emphasis on user choice and the corresponding social rights. This analysis shows the different ways to establish a care market and to introduce social rights. Second, the opening up of a care market does not imply a retreat of the state related to the mode of care delivery but instead provides a foundation for new state regulations with regard to quality, assessment, or user information. The analysis examines the newly defined state activities and the actors involved. Third, for the establishment of a care market and the new regulations of care delivery, the interplay of local and national state levels is decisive, notably the level of cohesiveness of policy development and the emphasis on decentralisation or centralisation of decision making. The analysis reveals the diverse interaction of local and national state levels in the countries compared.

GOVERNING THROUGH DELIVERY: CARE MARKETS AND USER CHOICE

In these countries, disparate measures have been introduced to increase the influence of the users on care provision. The care service infrastructure has been reorganised and new modes of service delivery have been developed to increase the voice of the individual user within care provision, including the establishment of user forums or councils aimed at enhancing the collective influence of the users. In this section, these different measures used to increase the user influence in our countries are analysed with regard to their shaping the policy development, and results, as well as the objectives embedded in care reforms in general, are discussed.

In this analysis, we discern three different forms of influence of the individual users: choice between service providers, choice related to the content of care provision, and choice between formal and informal care provision. These choices are at the centre of most reforms and related debates in the area (Lundsgaard, 2004a). In addition, we discuss different organisational forms to enhance the collective influence of the users. The introduction or new definition of social rights related to care and a restructured market–state relationship make the framework for the development of the changing concepts of the users. The analysis proceeds from the assumption that the interplay of local and national levels related to the policy subsystem of the care regimes and their general emphasis on the market or the state does much to define policies, their development, and their impact on home care. A summary of forms of user influence introduced in our countries is given in Table 7.1.

In the table, the forms of user influence are organised according to their availability, that is, whether they are regulated on a national level and generally available across the entire country and whether they are locally organised or a part of programmes targeted to specific groups. The criterion of availability is linked to further characteristics of the institutions, related primarily to the policy subsystem with their emphasis on centralisation or decentralisation and the level of cohesiveness. The characteristics of the policy subsystems thus provide the starting-point for the analysis of change. In all countries, efforts to enhance the influence of the individual users are strongly related to the introduction of a care market, with the opening up of care delivery for private for-profit and non-profit care providers. Only in a second step does the influence of the users came into the focus in the main by the introduction of freedom of choice among service providers, care offers, and formal or informal care.

In Germany, Japan and the Netherlands, care delivery is regulated by a national social insurance which provides the framework for a cohesive system of governance of formal care services. Despite different emphases in principle

Table 7.1 User influence: form and availability

Form of user influence	National level	Local level	Specific programme
Individual choice: service provider	Germany Japan Netherlands US	UK Sweden New Zealand	–
Individual choice: formal/informal care	Germany Netherlands	UK	Sweden
Individual choice: type of care offer	Germany Japan Netherlands US	UK	Sweden
Collective influence	Sweden	UK Sweden Germany	–

on the local or national level with regard to regulations in the three countries, in all the national level was decisive for the extension of care provision to private for-profit and non-profit care providers and the changing regulations with regard to user choice. With the introduction of the long-term care insurance (LTCI) in Germany in 1995 and Japan in 2001, a welfare mix of care providers was emphasised and care provision was opened to private providers. In both countries, the establishment of a care market was meant to further the quantitative expansion of care services and to create a variety of care offerings. While an expansion of service provision can be seen, investigations in Germany reveal that the providers offer essentially the same care packages regulated by the LTCI (Theobald, 2004). Also, in both countries choice of a service provider (with some local variations in Japan) and to a high degree the choice of the specific type of care service is possible on the basis of a maximum amount of money, set according to different levels of care needs.

In both Germany and Japan, user choice within formal care provision is widely accepted in society. While in Germany user choice constitutes an inherent characteristic of the health care system in general, in Japan the idea of maximising user choice is strongly related to the efforts to make the system more user friendly and thus overcome the cultural stigma against accepting help from outside the family (Ikegami et al., 2003; Rosenbrock and Gerlinger, 2004; Theobald, 2004). In contrast to Japan, the LTCI in Germany also enables freedom of choice between in-kind services and cash benefits to organise and pay for informal (principally family) care provision. With its goal of maintaining family care, the regulation is based on the family logic of care delivery embedded at least implicitly in the female part-time carer model. In Japan, the introduction of cash benefits was rejected because it was viewed as perpetuating the outdated traditional gender model which had to go and hampering the development of a care infrastructure (Karlsson et al., 2004: 28).

In the Netherlands, since the 1960s universally available home-based and residential services have been funded by the National Social Insurance for Exceptional Medical Risks. In contrast to Japan and Germany, where a new social insurance was introduced based on the principles of a care market and user choice, in the Netherlands the new developments were a part of the restructuring of care delivery. Since the 1990s, with its emphasis on increasing cost efficiency related to market mechanisms, more private for-profit providers have been established alongside the traditionally dominant private non-profit providers. Values such as patient orientation, user choice and service integration were explicitly incorporated only later (Knijn, 1998; Knijn and Verhagen, 2003; Kümpers, 2005). User choice among the different service providers is in principle possible in the entire country, but in practice it does not flourish because market pressures have meant that many providers have failed, thus making actual choice quite limited. Choice among different care offers is restricted. The types of formal care provision are decided on the basis of a needs assessment and a consideration of the available informal care sources (Pijl, 2003). The idea of user choice in the Netherlands is related to the personal budget programme introduced in the 1990s. The introduction of personal budgets is linked to the neo-liberal debate about the superiority of the market on the one hand and by debates by the client movement and liberal left on the other. In addition, the informal carer organisations saw personal budgets as a way to compensate for care giving. This explains the strength of the concept, which is applicable to the entire country and increasingly used (Tjadens and Duijnstee, 2000; Knijn and Verhagen, 2003; Kremer, 2005)

The UK and Sweden represent two care regimes which have traditionally been characterised by a public care provision financed by taxes and with a trend towards decentralisation of organised care provision at the local level. The relationship of the local and national levels, however, is quite different across these countries. While in Sweden decision making is highly decentralised based on a tradition of local democracy, in the UK efforts of decentralisation are part of a managerialist strategy under which decision making is often on a national level with responsibility for implementation delegated to the local level (Burau and Kröger, 2004; Rauch, 2005). In the UK since the 1990s, following from new public management initiatives a mixed economy of welfare was established based on an increasing share of private non-profit or for-profit providers. Between 1993 and 2004, the share of publicly provided home care decreased from 95 per cent of hours provided to only 31 per cent, with considerable local differences (Pavolini and Ranci, 2006).

Initially, the introduction of market mechanisms through competition among providers focused on cost efficiency, but the issue of the influence of the users has often been a byproduct, especially at the level of policies (Means et al., 2003; Baggot et al., 2005; Kümpers, 2005). This has slightly changed with the New Labour government, which has put a more explicit focus on user choice under which *consumerism* is presented as a generic principle for public services (Vidler and Clarke, 2005). However, with a lack of adequate funding and implementation at the local level, especially related to social care, it is unclear what will eventuate in practice. Since 2000, direct payments have been available as an option for the elderly, which grants them a certain basic amount with their choice as to whether to spend it on formal or informal care provision. Direct payments have emerged from user struggles to exercise control over the forms and relationships of support, particularly from the disabled movement. New Labour has now extended the principle of direct payments to older people (Clarke, nd). Despite the rhetoric of the national government, however, the scheme has only very limited availability at the municipality level (Ungerson, 2003; Lundsgaard, 2004a).

At the beginning of the 1990s, in Sweden care provision was opened up for private providers at a national level based on the right of the municipalities to decide on the issue on their own. In 2004 about 10 per cent of the hours of social care for the elderly aged 65 years and older are delivered by private, mainly for-profit service providers (SOS, 2005a). In general, the establishment of private for-profit providers was strongly related to price competition between providers, aimed at a more cost-efficient service provision (Edebalk and Svensson, 2005). Only in a second stage was user choice between service providers introduced in 10 Swedish municipalities, for the most part around Stockholm (ibid.). Despite the objective of more cost-efficient services, an evaluation of the National Board of Health and Welfare shows a slightly higher cost increase in municipalities with competition between service providers than those without (SOS, 2004 in Vabo, 2005). The opening up of care provision for private care providers locally varies considerably due to the right of the municipalities to decide on the issue (Brodin, 2005; SOS, 2005a). Social care provision is a core activity of the Swedish welfare state and the variations between the municipalities reflect different ideas on the role of the market and the state within social care provision (Brodin, 2005).

In Sweden, service provision is decided on the basis of a needs assessment under the Law on Social Services where care services should be provided according to the wishes of the individual care recipient (SOS, 2004). More user choice between different types of care options is available within two programmes for specific target groups. Regulated by a national law, people with severe functional impairments are granted a personal budget to decide on their own care provision (Szebehely, 2005). The introduction of freedom of choice between formal and informal care provision is based on the demands of the disabled people's movement (Edebalk and Svensson, 2005). In some municipalities, elderly people at a certain age and with a low level of needs are granted a small amount of funds which they can use freely for different services (Hjalmarson, 2006). Investigations into the issue of user choice in the Nordic countries reveal that elderly care recipients are more interested in deciding on the content and conduct of daily care provision than choosing between service providers (Edebalk and Svensson, 2005; Vabo, 2005).

In contrast to the other countries compared here, the US and New Zealand have traditionally allowed private for-profit care providers to be involved in care delivery. In the US this follows a highly fragmented and decentralised provision of formal care with an emphasis on private care, and in New Zealand it is linked to a mix of publicly owned home health services and private and voluntary agencies (Stone, 2000; New Zealand Ministry of Health, 2002b; Centres for Medicare and Medicaid Services, 2003a). Recently in New Zealand a more centralised and cohesive form of formal care provision has emerged. Since the early 1990s, public policy has supported a philosophy of 'ageing in place', a key strategy of which includes increasing public expenditure and public control on home care and support services (New Zealand Ministry of Health, 2002b). While traditionally users have had little say in care provision and despite little public debate, under these initiatives user choice among service providers and to a lesser extent increased opportunities to decide on the content of the delivered service are being emphasised. However, freedom of choice between service providers due to market constraints is available only in large populated areas. In the US, users have a choice both as to service providers and service options. Objectives to increase user choice are largely related to cost containment, with the unproven assumption that competition among providers will lower costs.

Besides measures to enhance individual user choice and the influence of the users on care provision, approaches for a collective empowerment of the users can be found in the European countries compared. In the UK under the National Health Service and the 1990 Community and Care Act, the local authorities are required to develop community care plans in consultation with service users and informal carers. This has stimulated the spread of local older people's forums, although there remains considerable local variation regarding the scope of consultation with these groups (Ginn and Arber, 1999) in relation to health care, the community health councils founded in 1974 traditionally represented the main institutionalised form of collective influence. The 2001 Health and Social Care Act abolished the community health councils and replaced them with patient and public involvement forums that operate under the auspices of a new national organisation, the Commission for Patient and Public Involvement in Health (Baggot et al., 2005).

In the Netherlands, the governance structure in both health and social care is based on corporatism but also includes consumer groups (Exter et al., 2004). Under the umbrella of the Dutch Federation of Patients and Consumers, such groups are members of the Health Insurance Board which is responsible for the management of the two social insurance schemes as well as the advisory body, the Council for Public Health and Health Care. In contrast to the UK and the Netherlands, in Germany approaches to enhance the influence of user groups within the health or long-term care system are in their infancy (Sachverständigenrat für die Konzertierte Aktion im Gesundheitswesen, 2001/2002). However, efforts have already been undertaken at the local level to enhance the influence of pensioners in the political system. Since the 1970s, municipal-level senior citizen councils that can be involved in the organisation of services have been voluntarily established. The actual power of senior citizen councils depends to a great extent on the local conditions and opportunities which vary across municipalities (Naegele, 1999). A general trend can be observed in Sweden to increase the influence of pensioners on political decisions on a local and a national level. Since the 1970s, senior citizen councils have existed at the local level and since the 1990s at the national level. At a local level, the power of the councils varies and is dependent on the expertise of the members. At the national level the councils strengthened their influence over decisions during the 1990s, as evidenced by the introduction of a law concerning maximum fees within formal care provision (Feltenius, 2004).

GOVERNING THROUGH FUNDING: SOCIAL RIGHTS AND USER CHOICE

Different measures to increase user choice in care provision are not limited to privately financed services. The measures are very often covered by public funding based on social insurances or taxes (Lundsgaard, 2004a). The implementation of user choice within a public funding system does not imply necessarily that freedom of choice is available for all users and with regard to all types of services. In this chapter the tensions between the state and the market logic, that is, public or private funding of services, are analysed. The tensions between public or private funding concern the groups among the users that are eligible to receive publicly funded services, the range of services covered, and the level of public funding. Eligibility criteria related to social rights, funding principles of benefits, and the range of in-kind services publicly covered determine the availability of user choice for certain user groups. In this section the relationship between user choice on the one hand

and the quality of social rights and different funding principles on the other are compared. Thus tensions between the concept of freedom of choice and the concept of equality defined as equal access of the users to different types of user choice are discussed.

The analysis proceeds from the assumption that the quality of social rights, that is, eligibility criteria and funding principles linked to the different care regimes, define the relationship between equality and user choice. Care regimes oriented towards universalism and a comprehensive funding of care services more often provide the basis for the employment of user choice for different groups of people in need of care. In contrast, user choice is more often accentuated in care regimes with limited social rights. Table 7.2 provides an overview on forms of user choice and their relationship to the quality of social rights.

Table 7.2 User choice and funding

Form of user choice	Comprehensive/ universal	Basic funding/ universal	Means tested
Service provider	Sweden Japan Netherlands	Germany	UK New Zealand US
Type of care offer	Sweden Japan Netherlands	Germany	UK US
Formal/informal care	Sweden Netherlands	Germany	UK

According to the quality of social rights, these countries can be divided into three types which apply for all three comparisons made (see Table 7.2). Within the means-tested care regimes of the UK, New Zealand and the US, service provision is often targeted only at people below a certain income limit. Characteristic of these three countries is a mixed structure of means-tested and universally available services that have changed in the course of the restructurings. In contrast, two care regimes oriented towards public services, Sweden and the Netherlands, offer a universal and comprehensive funding of care services. Meanwhile Japan and Germany, representing the subsidiary care regime, have moved in two opposite directions with the introduction of their LTCI plans. In Japan, care services are universal accessible and comprehensive to needs, while in Germany the universal available benefits cover a basic provision only and have to be complemented by informal care or further privately paid care.

In the Netherlands, Sweden and Japan, user choice is offered through a wide range of care services and care options collectively covered to create a comprehensive care arrangement. User choice may be limited with regard to two respects. First, the level and construction of fees and the definition of family responsibility may hamper the use of care services as a whole or of a specific type of service. In Sweden since the 1990s, the use of services with regard to minor needs – housekeeping activities or support to social activities – has declined. This decline can partly be explained by high fees and the increasing consideration of family care resources (Szebehely, 1999a, b, 2000). Recently in some municipalities, programmes or model projects have been established that provide the elderly over a certain age with the opportunity of a limited number of hours of home care service which they can use freely. Evaluations show that due to high user fees, the demand for such services has been less than expected (Hjalmarson, 2006).

In the Netherlands, high user fees inhibit the use of some in-kind services because high co-payments mean that some potential users may not be able to afford them. Furthermore, during the needs assessment informal care resources that limit the scope of granted care services are considered. The carer organisations have criticised this practice and argued that in many cases the informal carers are obliged to do more than they are able to do (Pijl, 2003). Personal budgets are collectively funded on the same level as in-kind services. There are no distinct profiles of care users preferring cash benefits or in-kind services in the Netherlands (Miltenburg, 2004). Also with regard to personal budgets, high user fees and the consideration of informal family care limit choices in care provision. Current debates related to demands of cost containment stress the limits of the scope of social insurance by increasing co-payments and tightening up on the rules for needs assessment (Visser-Jansen and Knipscheer, 2004).

In Japan, cost-containment policies centre on the idea of moving from residential care to home care, while the money provided by the LTCI should provide the means to establish a universal and user-friendly care infrastructure (Japan Ministry of Health, Labour and Welfare, 2004b). Within the framework of the LTCI, a certain amount of money is granted according to needs for the purchase of in-kind services with freedom of choice between services providers and different types of services. Co-payments of 10 per cent are calculated which can be waived by municipalities for beneficiaries after means testing. In principle, choice is funded collectively; however, the way the fees are constructed influences user choice. The level of 10 per cent set for co-payments is independent of the type of services, and because of higher co-payments for personal than for practical help, less personal help is purchased. In practice, therefore, freedom of choice with regard to personal care is concentrated in beneficiaries with higher incomes (Campbell and Ikegami, 2003).

Also in Japan, the Netherlands and Sweden, user choice between service providers is linked to an opening up of care provision for private for-profit providers and the introduction of market principles. In all three countries, due to market principles in service provision the private service offerings have either vanished or are only rarely available at the periphery. Higher costs of service provision which may not be compensated and the low demand at the margins make service provision for-profit providers unprofitable (for Sweden, see, for example, Edebalk and Svensson, 2005; for Japan, see Noguchi and Shimizutani, 2005).

Within the framework of the LTCI in Germany, choice among service providers and different types of service options as well as between formal and informal care is in principle possible but in practice it is impeded due to the level of funding. The choice between formal and informal care provision is influenced by the principle of basic funding only. Most care recipients prefer cash benefits, however, with discernible social differences. Beneficiaries in the upper middle class choose in-kind services instead of cash benefits more often than recipients of the lower or lower middle classes (Blinkert and Klie, 1999; Klie and Blinkert, 2002). Under basic funding, the use of in-kind services necessitates either the purchase of further paid services, even on the grey market, or the provision of further informal care which (also) encourages beneficiaries with a lower income to vote for cash benefits (Blinkert and Klie, 1999; Klie and Blinkert, 2002).

In contrast to the care regimes discussed above, the care regimes in the US, New Zealand and the UK are oriented not towards universalism but include elements of means testing with regard to home care as a whole or to specific areas. Varied developments with regard to social rights to care and the introduction of more user choice can be observed in these countries. In New Zealand, paralleling the increasing opportunities for more user choice, care services are more often universally available, thus extending the range of opportunities of choice for an increasing proportion of the population. Since the 1990s, public policy has supported a philosophy of ageing in place, a key strategy which includes increasing public expenditure on home care and support services. The government partially or fully subsidises a wide range of home care services with eligibility and level of services determined by needs assessment. This makes for a mixed service infrastructure where some care offers are universally available after means testing or based on voluntary organisations (New Zealand Ministry of Health, 2002b; New Zealand Ministry for Senior Citizens, 2001; New Zealand Ministry of Social Policy, 2001). Means testing for some types of long-term care skews the distribution towards the lower strata, especially to those who have not saved for retirement. In general, a trend can be seen to phase out means testing. Care services are traditionally provided by a mix of public, private for-profit and non-profit providers with user choice of providers only in the populated areas.

In the UK a more contradictory development of care services can be found. The (rhetorical) emphasis on user choice, as well as the introduction of different measures to increase the opportunity for user preference combined with a lack of funding from the national level, has led to considerable local dissimilarities with regard to implementation. More decisive for the prospect of user choice is the health and social care divide with regard to funding principles. Here shifts in the health and social care following the introduction of the internal care market in the early 1990s are decisive for access to different types of services. This has led to a hollowing out of entitlements to universal tax-funded health services, together with the redefinition of care needs such as means-tested social services and high co-payments (Glendinning, 1998; Lewis, 2001). In fact, freedom of choice has been reduced for some groups within community care with regard to some types of services. Care services in the community are primarily available to those who have both a high level of need and whose income and assets are below a certain level. For the rest, majority care is supplied by family, neighbours and the private and voluntary sector (Baldock, 2003). The introduction of free personal care in Scotland led to a debate about the extent of public funding of home care services. Among other factors this provided the background for a Royal Commission, which looked into future options for the public funding of home care (OECD, 2005b).

In the US, the idea of user choice is assumed; however, social rights under the two tax-funded public systems, Medicare and Medicaid, limit access to certain defined groups of users and additionally restrict the scope of available services. Under Medicare, only basic health services are covered for older people, with virtually no support given for home care (Centers for Medicare and Medicaid Services, 2003a). Only after means testing do directed Medicaid programmes pick up the total costs of formal home care. Moreover, under these programmes care recipients must follow state packages with restricted choices. In contrast, most home care is privately funded by the growing long-term care insurance industry. This situation is especially difficult for the lower middle class, which gets no support at all but is not affluent enough to purchase or organise private home care.

GOVERNING THROUGH RULES: NEW REGULATIONS AND THE INTERPLAY OF LOCAL AND NATIONAL LEVELS

The changing role of the user, notably the emphasis on user choice and social rights related to care, has led to the introduction of further measures related to the access to benefits or services and the delivery of care services. The exercise of choice between different service providers and service offers presupposes an informed user, that is, a care user able to gather and assess information. The introduction of social rights is linked to a definition of collective care needs and formalised assessment procedures which aim at guaranteeing a fair and equal access to care provision for different groups among people in need of care. The establishment of a care market strengthened efforts to improve the care quality.

The different activities with regard to the provision of information, definitions of assessment procedures, and measures related to quality assurance have required the introduction of laws and regulations by the state. In our countries, regulations and laws which include the definition of the involvement of further non-state actors have been established by the state at national and local levels. This requires the analysis of the interaction of regulations and implementation on different levels of state activities and the role taken by non-state actors. This section proceeds from the assumption that the policy subsystems with their characteristic interrelationships among national and local state levels as well as the state and non-state actors involved in care provision in general explain the mode of introduction of the different measures. Decisive for the introduction of the regulations is the level of cohesiveness between the levels. Furthermore, within a cohesive policy subsystem the emphasis on the national and local levels may change for the assorted areas considered. Table 7.3 organises our countries according to the area of regulation and the level involved.

Table 7.3 Areas and level of regulation

Areas of regulation	National/strong universal	Local universal	Specific programmes
Information	New Zealand Japan Sweden Germany	US	New Zealand
Assessment	Germany New Zealand Japan Netherlands	Sweden UK US	–
Quality assurance	Germany UK Japan	Sweden New Zealand US	–

Investigations into the role of home care users have revealed the difficulties for many elderly users to act as rational consumers on a market and to take advantage of the different care offers and the opportunities of choice (Glendinning, 1998; Sachverständigenrat für die Konzertierte Aktion im Gesundheitswesen, 2001/2002; Edebalk and Svensson, 2005). Against this background, the countries compared have introduced an array of measures to enable care users to have a more informed choice. With the possible exception of the highly fragmented policy subsystem of the US, the national level is decisive for the introduction of regulations related to the provision of information. Even the Home Health Quality Initiative, which aims to empower consumers with quality of care information to make more informed decisions, began as a test programme in eight states (US Department of Health and Human Services, 2003).

In Sweden under the national Social Service Act, beneficiaries have the right to information on different types of support and help available on the municipal level as a precondition for an individualised care provision (SOS, 2004). In addition, at the municipal level after an assessment the assessors are obliged to provide the beneficiaries with information on the different service providers (Edebalk and Svensson, 2005). In New Zealand within the framework of ageing in place initiatives organised at a national level, the assessors are to provide information on service providers to every user after an assessment at District Health Board level (New Zealand Ministry of Health, 2002b). In Japan within the LTCI framework, the assessors at the Long-Term Care Approval Board provide complete programme information after an assessment of the person. In Germany, according to the 2002 law on Quality Assurance and Customer Protection, the care insurance funds are obliged to compile lists on options and prices of the different providers in the area and make them available to care users, while the care users are expected to gather information on service providers on their own.

The Netherlands provides a more specific case for involvement at the national level because the debate on a national level has not yet resulted in any regulation. With the introduction of personal budgets on a national level, an obligatory case management was rejected, leaving to the care users or their relatives the responsibility of organising their own care services. As a result, user groups and self-help groups of budget holders are actively involved in counselling prospective users. Meanwhile, the necessity of an obligatory case management among the personal budget programme for certain groups is being discussed (Klie, 2004).

Social or citizenship rights to care are strongly related to the issue of equal access to care provision according to needs. Eligibility criteria and assessment procedures are aimed at guaranteeing equal access to care provision for different user groups. In their cross-national comparison, Blackman et al.

(2001) confirm that the establishment of a formalised assessment procedure linked to strict eligibility criteria is a decisive step towards fair access to social care services.

In the UK, Sweden and the US, the local levels are responsible for the definition of assessment procedures. In Sweden and the UK, the interplay of state and local laws or regulations reflect the more cohesive policy subsystem, while in the US the local regulations are developed without a common national framework. In Sweden and the UK, a legal right to a needs assessment can be found at the national level. In the latter, the introduction of the rights to a needs assessment and the provision of a charter to equitable access went hand in hand with a great emphasis on care/case management as a means to move from service to needs-led provision of high-quality care (Glendinning, 1998; Means et al., 2003). In Sweden, the Social Service Act and related recommendations prescribe an integral assessment as the precondition for an individualised care arrangement and high-quality care (SOSFS, 1998; SOS, 2004). In both countries, the municipalities are responsible for the establishment of assessment procedures, which in both countries results in considerable variation regarding access to services (Glendinning, 1998; Trydegard, 2003). In the US, assessment criteria are introduced at a local level, with considerable differences among states and localities.

In Germany, New Zealand, Japan and the Netherlands, regulations with regard to assessment procedures are defined more strictly on a national level. In the Netherlands, comparable assessments have been introduced at a regional level where agencies assess the needs of the individuals. After approval by the social insurance, the needs assessment provides the basis for formal and informal care provision. This has resulted in a needs-led service provision. In New Zealand, national levels of care dependency are defined as a basis for an assessment. In addition, ageing in place initiatives include small steps towards a uniform assessment system through the imposition of initial guidelines.

Within the framework of their respective LTCI plans, in Japan and Germany levels of care needs are defined for the entire country relative to the maximum amount of money available. In addition, in Germany the law prescribes that the associations of the care insurance funds and the medical services of the health insurance funds are responsible for the development of national assessment procedures. In Germany, the idea of equality is strongly related to a fair assessment, that is, with the same level of needs the applicants should be assigned the same level of care dependency. Against this background, two issues of inequality – regional and social – have been widely discussed. Despite efforts for a uniform assessment procedure for the entire country, there are still differences between the federal states (*Bundesländer*) with regard to the proportion of beneficiaries among the elderly aged 65 years and older

(Federal Statistical Office, 2005a). Furthermore, a comparison of assessment results of the social LTCI which covers approximately 90 per cent of the population and the (mandatory) private long-term care insurance which covers 10 per cent of the population (for the most part the upper middle class) reveals that the applications within the framework of the private insurance are less often rejected and they are more often assigned to higher care-dependency levels, despite the use of the same criteria (Bundesministerium für Gesundheit, 2004).

The tension between the introduction of market mechanisms such as access of private for-profit providers on the one hand and the ongoing public responsibility and funding of care services on the other, supports the introduction of measures designed to ensure the quality of care provision. In all countries compared here, the national level is involved in quality assurance regulations, however, with considerable differences as to the form of these regulations and the level of discretion granted local officials. In Germany, Japan and the UK, strong national regulations are common. In the UK, national quality standards have been introduced and the National Care Standard Commission was created. In Japan, the introduction of the LTCI elevated the definition of quality standards to the national level; however, implementation and control is delegated to the regional or municipal level (Japan Ministry of Health, 2004b). This latter pattern reflects the decentralised but cohesive policy subsystem in Japan.

Related to the developments since the introduction of the LTCI, in 2002 the Quality Assurance and Consumer Protection Act came into effect in Germany at the national level. It prescribes actors' responsibilities and quality assurance measures valid for the entire country. The law obliges all service providers to introduce quality assurance management and conduct regular controls. On behalf of the care insurance funds, the medical service of the health care insurances is entitled to supervise the care quality of the service providers (Bundesministerium für Gesundheit, 2004). The involvement of further non-state actors, such as the insurance funds or the medical service, reflects the general characteristics of Germany's decentralised policy subsystem.

In New Zealand, Sweden and the US, the regulations at the national level are less strict, with the weakest types of national regulations found in the highly fragmented and decentralised US care system. In the US, the states are only required to certify to the federal government that they have established adequate quality assurance methods. In New Zealand, national-level guidelines have been worked out that are used by many local-level service providers to develop internal quality assurance programmes. In addition, under ageing in place initiatives, quality expectations are written into service contracts at District Health Board level (New Zealand Ministry of Health, 2006). In

Sweden under the Social Service Act at the national level, care provision of a 'good quality' is stipulated. In addition, recommendations worked out by the National Board of Health and Welfare (Socialstyrelsen) describe in greater detail the areas of quality work, adequate measures of quality, and expected municipal responsibility. However, it remains up to the municipality to decide on the measures needed to ensure or improve the care quality (SOSFS, 1998; SOS, 2004).

With the exception of the highly fragmented US care system, in all these countries one can see a changing interplay of policy development between the national and local levels, with new types of national regulations introduced to improve the quality of care and the condition of the care users. On the basis of laws, guidelines and standards, an administrative view on care quality has been established. Critical research on users reveals the widely diverse perspectives of the users on quality, fashioned in the course of interactions in daily caring situations (Hojlund, 2005; Zeman, 2005). Simultaneously, the emergence of new demands on elderly care impedes individual-oriented care provision as a basis for a good care quality and provides a decisive starting-point for the development.

CASE STUDIES

In the countries compared here, the changing conceptions of users have been introduced in the light of a new mix of market and state principles in care provision and a new definition of social rights. The UK and Germany are selected as countries representing two different modes of developments. In the UK, the changes have occurred more gradually and within the framework of a means-tested care regime. In Germany, the introduction of the LTCI regulated the risk of frailty based on the social insurance principle and brought about significant changes for the social rights related to care, as well as a new mix of market and state principles. The defined regulations, however, signalled a significant departure from the German social insurance tradition. This comparison reveals the policy development within the two countries and thus explains the country-specific mix of state and market principles and how it has been established.

Changing Definitions of Care Users in the UK: The Interplay between Market and State Logics

The UK represents an interesting case of changing definitions of care users. This is one of the countries where the logic of the market with its idea of freedom of choice is most evident. At the same time, developments at the policy level are characterised by changing conceptions of user choice, increasingly moving from reforms of service delivery and the involvement of care users in service development to more direct forms of user choice such as direct payments to carers. This shift has been accompanied by a gradual introduction of basic social rights associated with the logic of the state. However, the co-existence of both sets of logics is characterised by tensions in the broader context of a means-tested care regime.

In the public debate in the UK, the issues around care users and their influence is strongly related to the introduction of market mechanisms in health and social care through competition among providers and a focus on cost efficiency (see Baldock, 1998). The market logic frames care users as consumers who have freedom of choice. Initially, as part of the introduction of the internal market in health and social care in the early 1990s, policies defined choice especially as choices in relation to the organisation and delivery of formal care services. The assumption seemed to be that changes in service provision would increase the choice of users more or less by default. In addition, particularly in relation to health care, there were individual initiatives that explicitly aimed at strengthening the involvement of users as such, for example, the 1992 Local Voices initiatives and the 1996 Patient Partnership initiative (Baggot et al., 2005).

In comparison, the New Labour government has had a more explicit concern with care users as consumers as part of its focus on the modernisation of public services (Clarke, nd). Indeed, New Labour presents 'consumerism' as a generic organising principle for public services (Vidler and Clarke, 2005). Thus user involvement is meant to become an integral part of the running of welfare services (Baggot et al., 2005). This has to be seen against the background of the widespread critique of the effect of Conservative reforms on public services, as well as consumers' attempts to include both the desire for better services and the doubt about the capacity of governments to deliver (Vidler and Clarke, 2005). The more explicit focus on users as consumers goes hand in hand with more extensive policy initiatives that point to an emerging interchange between the logics of the market and the state with its focus on social rights. The government has played a very central role in the public debate about care users and their influence, especially under the New Labour government. The debates here centre around how processes of modernisation (such as the increasing individualisation of society) require the adaptation of welfare services and more specifically the strengthening of users (and formerly only citizens) as consumers (Clarke, nd).

In their study of health consumer groups, Baggot et al. (2005) suggest that the introduction of the internal market in the early 1990s (and especially the adverse consequences the reform was feared to have), together with the tight timetable for consultation, encouraged the formation of coalitions of user groups. In relation to home care, for example, Carers' Alliance UK was key and aimed at making a private problem into a public issue. Similarly, Barnes characterises the 1990s as a period of consolidation: 'Carers were "discovered" by policy-makers and were urged to "come out" by organizations such as the Carers National Association (CAN) and by local carers' organizations' (2001: 195).

A forerunner organisation for single women and their dependants had campaigned for support, especially in financial terms, of women carers and had achieved the payment of the Invalid Care Allowance directly to carers. Over the years, the focus of the organisation was broadened to include all kinds of carers. This development helped to establish the identity of a carer and for carers as a social group to become the subject of public policies. Here the gradual move away from concerns about the financial support of carers (especially through the allowance) towards a focus on the broader recognition of the role of carers is also indicative. Furthermore, the campaigning work of the present organisation, Carers UK, is very much based on a social rights approach typical of the state logic. In fact, the organisation describes itself as at the forefront of securing legal rights for carers (Carers UK, nd). Carers UK has supported many recent policy initiatives that introduce basic social rights for carers, such as the right to request direct payment (Carers UK, 2001, 2005). Not surprisingly, the organisation is critical of the fact that the government makes little additional funding available because this potentially weakens social rights in practice.

The implementation of new definitions of users as consumers has occurred in a means-tested care regime where the state support for formal care and more recently also informal care has tended to be limited to those groups most in need. In terms of the substance of corresponding policies, this has meant that the market logic with its emphasis on freedom of choice has been dominant, while substantive social rights (as typical of the state logic) have tended to be less developed. Although this is changing to some extent, the overall balance between market and state logics remains intact. In relation to specific policies, this leads to a number of tensions.

As suggested above, when the internal market was first introduced in the early 1990s the restructuring of service provision and the involvement of care users in service development were seen as important levers for the exercise of user choice. In respect of the first aspect, changes have meant that services respond better to individual needs, allow for different options and concentrate on those with the greatest need (Means et al., 2003). Concerning the second aspect, measures include user involvement in the process of assessment and the development of community care plans as well as the introduction of complaints procedures (Barnes et al., 1999). Indeed, the provision of care services has been characterised by a gradual but clear shift from the public to the private non-profit/for-profit sector (Means et al., 2003). At the same time there has been a strong emphasis on care/case management as a means of moving from service to needs-led provision of care (Glendinning, 1998). This in fact means 'choice by proxy', and as such put limits on user choice. Yet the role of case managers as gatekeepers is central in a care regime where public support is meant to be limited and targeted.

Subsequently, the support of informal care has become a central focus for the development of user choice. Since the early 1990s, government policies have acknowledged the contribution of informal carers to care arrangements. The 1996 Carers (Recognition and Services) Act introduced the right to needs assessment, but made no provisions to support carers in practice. This changed in part with the Carers and Disabled Children Act in 2000, when local authorities were allowed to introduce 'direct payments for carers'. This became a statutory duty with the 2004 Carers (Equal Opportunities) Act. Significantly, adequate matching funds have not followed, and the support of informal carers therefore remains highly resource dependent and choice therefore remains limited (Barnes et al., 1999). It is also indicative that the numbers of carers receiving this type of benefit is very low. According to Lundsgaard (2004a), in 2003 only 0.04 per cent of all people aged 65 or over received direct payments. Similarly, Ungerson (2003) suggests that in 2002 just over 1000 older people were in receipt of such direct payments. Although the substantive support of informal carers is often symbolic, developments since the mid-1990s have been characterised by the introduction of basic social rights, and the logic of the state increasingly complements the logic of the market.

In summary, in the UK care users have become more central to the public debate, and policy initiatives since the mid-1990s have introduced a number of basic social rights for care users. As a result, care users enjoy more and increasingly direct choices, although choice often remains limited and uncertain, reflecting funding constraints and strong variation across localities.

The Introduction of the LTCI in Germany: A New Balance between State and Market Logic in a Social Insurance System

In Germany, with the introduction of the LTCI in 1995/96, the role of users in care provision and social rights changed significantly. The incentive for the establishment of this new pillar within the German social insurance system was provided by the increasing costs for residential care which had to be funded by the municipalities after means testing (Ostner, 1998; Campell and Morgan, 2005). The introduction of a social insurance to regulate a social risk corresponds to the German social insurance tradition. Despite this, basic regulations mandated by the law brought about a significant departure from the German social security tradition with regard to the mix of state and market principles and the quality of social rights.

The changes introduced by the LTCI involve both the mode of delivery and funding of long-term care services. Competition between service providers and freedom of choice for users are basic characteristics of the German health care system (Rosenbrock and Gerlinger, 2004). Within the framework of the LTCI based on the idea of market superiority, both principles were newly defined and assigned a fresh role within care provision. Before the introduction of the LTCI, primarily non-profit care providers and to a smaller extent private for-profit providers delivered long-term care. Based on the principle of subsidiarity, the non-profit providers as the main care providers took a privileged position and could receive different types of state subsidies. With the introduction of the LTCI, both non-profit and for-profit providers are to deliver care on equal terms. The regulations aimed at enabling competition on equal terms between both types of care providers, thus ensuring more cost-efficient prices in daily care delivery as well as achieving an increase of freedom of choice for the users between care providers. The law reflected the increasing involvement of private for-profit providers, justified on the basis of more cost-efficient prices since the 1980s (Landenberger, 1994; Meyer, 1996; Schmidt, 2002).

The establishment of a care market on equal terms for private for-profit and non-profit service providers and the principle of freedom of choice were defined as the foundation of the development of a care infrastructure. The demand for care services and different care options by the users became the basic rationale for the expansion of care services, while social planning to achieve a comprehensive infrastructure was defined as negligible (Landenberger, 1994). In contrast to the opening up of the care market, the neglect of social planning by state authorities sparked an intense debate by the actors involved (see Meyer, 1996). While the Liberal Party (in government with the Christian-Democratic party at that time) emphasised the role of the market, the Christian-Democratic party and notably the Social Democratic party suggested a more decisive role for social planning for the establishment of a care infrastructure. Within the government coalition, the liberals prevailed with their market-oriented principles because they accepted the establishment of a social insurance only under the premise of exerting a strong influence on the regulations.

In the last round of negotiation between the coalition of the federal government and the Social Democratic Party representing the majority in the Bundesrat (the second federal chamber composed of representatives of the governments of the federal states or *Bundesländer*) the emphasis on the role of user demand, cost-efficient prices and competition as principles for the development of the care infrastructure were confirmed. However, the obligation of the federal states to subsidise investments provided space for social planning to some degree. In fact, after the introduction of the law the expansion of the home care infrastructure occurred mainly within the logic of the market. Care services in principle are available on demand across the country, with even an oversupply of service providers in the big cities. In contrast, the goal to establish diverse care offerings based on the demand of the users has not been achieved, and the service providers offer the same regulated care services almost everywhere (Theobald, 2004).

Based on the market principle and the freedom of choice, in Germany, therefore, users had a significant role in the development of a care infrastructure. However, the level of public funding for long-term care services defined by the law questions whether the defined user rights, particularly their freedom of choice, are underpinned by corresponding social rights. Within the framework of the Health Care Insurance, based on the decision of a medical doctor, in principle unlimited health care services are granted according to health needs. At the beginning of the debate on the introduction of the LTCI, most of the actors involved argued for a funding of long-term care comparable to the level of the health care insurance (see Meyer, 1996). In the course of the debate, however, the more economically oriented actors gradually prevailed. In particular the cost increase, the so-called 'cost explosion' within the framework of the health care insurance, was used as the most significant argument against full coverage of care needs. During the final negotiations between the Christian-Democratic and Liberal federal government and the Social Democratic Party, the leading party of the Bundesrat, they agreed that the insurance should provide only basic funding, that is, defined benefits on different levels which do not cover all care needs. The non-profit associations, which view themselves as advocates for the users and which are responsible for most care services, accepted the principle of a basic funding only at the end and claimed success (even against the municipalities as financiers) in gaining the availability of supplementary social assistance benefits to cover fully the care needs for beneficiaries with lower incomes, after means testing.

In contrast to the health insurance, the final regulation of the LTCI still defines the risk of frailty as an individual risk with the social insurance granting basic funding only, that is, the costs are only partly covered by the social insurance and have to be supplemented by private means or informal care delivery. Furthermore, the regulations do not consider the economic situation of the users since every beneficiary receives the same level of benefit independent of the income situation or assets. According to Landenberger (1994) the regulations indicate a reduction of the social insurance tradition to a basic funding system without any elements of solidarity. Since the introduction of the LTCI, the decision to cover only basic costs for services impedes the use of formal care services by members of the lower classes, who therefore become more dependent on informal care provision (Blinkert and Klie, 1999; Klie and Blinkert, 2002).

In conclusion, with the introduction of the LTCI the role of the user of home care in Germany has been drastically changed under a newly regulated care infrastructure oriented towards market principles. The quality of the social rights related to the insurance limits user choice. Despite the universal orientation of the law, the principle of basic funding only impedes the use of care services, especially for the members of the lower classes.

NOTE

1. In Estonia and Italy, the use of care services is very limited and discussions on the changing role of the users or user choice are only marginal. Therefore, neither country is taken into account in the analysis of this chapter.

8. Home care governance: mapping out convergences and divergences

This chapter returns to the comparative policy context of home care. It discusses the issues and tensions that underlie governing arrangements regarding the funding, provision and rules of home care across the various countries. It summarises the findings concerning the logics and instruments of home care governance introduced in Chapter 1, and discusses what we have learned about patterns and differences in home care governance across these countries. It also summarises what we see as the most crucial factors surrounding the formal/informal mix that comprises home care identified in the substantive chapters. What mix of public and private and formal and informal? This chapter also discusses the extent to which these countries are dealing with the challenges raised by home care and how the widely disparate policies reflect the institutional and value differences across the countries. Finally, it examines whether governance initiatives across the countries are leading to a policy convergence in home care or illustrate continued divergence.

This book has demonstrated that home care is a multifaceted pursuit that includes a wide range of tasks which transcend the distinction between formal services and informal relationships. While the formal services dimension links home care governance to the dynamics of policy making, informal care ties home care governance to the wider family and gender structures in society. Home care can be delivered by trained health and social care professionals or by untrained paid helpers, family or friends. Home care is a difficult policy area to study because it blurs the boundary between public and private life that is evident in more traditional policy areas. Although many home services are provided through an array of public and private organisational structures, a considerable amount of home care is informal and thus traditionally outside the purview of public control.

In order to account for the complexity of home care, we have focused on the broader concept of governance instead of the more conventionally studied public policy. We argue that while established policy institutions are important, in order to understand home care governance we must scrutinise all the relevant institutions and ideas, including those outside government. Therefore we have included in our analysis (sector-specific) social and political institutions as well as broader institutional arrangements such as the welfare state and the political system. Finally, in terms of ideas we looked at culturally embedded traditions, beliefs and attitudes and the changing nature of ideas relating to home care in these countries.[1]

In relation to Figure 1.1, we suggested that there are two routes to the governance of home care, a direct route and an indirect one where the policy process acts so as to shape it. Although we argue for a comprehensive analysis of the varied logics, the fundamental intervening variable is public policy. Home care policy was defined as those courses of action or non-action proposed or taken by a government that impact on the financing, delivery or rule of home care services. While attention logically focused on governments, however, the inclusion of the other logics of governance (including the actions by private and voluntary organisations, the market and the family) were found to have a crucial impact on home care governance. Moreover, we found that in some countries, state non-action in the home care arena until recently has been a more common approach than action. It is also clear from our analysis that home care is interconnected with social and economic policy in general, and therefore cannot be understood in isolation from social welfare, health, unemployment, poverty, housing and general economic policies. That is what makes studying home care governance especially demanding.

In the light of the complexity of governing home care uncovered in Chapters 2 and 3, this analysis has offered comparative insights as to the governance of home care under a wide variety of institutional and value contexts. We suggest that cross-cultural studies are helpful both in illustrating the commonalities of problems and variables across countries and for taking into consideration the full array of options. While home care governance is seen as unique to each nation, since all countries are facing comparable dynamics of demographic and social changes we cannot underestimate the globalisation of problems and of potential solutions.

HOME CARE ACROSS NATIONS

The data on long-term care presented in Table 4.2 demonstrated that long-term care at present represents a relatively small part of public spending (around 0.5 per cent of GDP or less in our countries) and an even smaller portion of private spending in the form of out-of-pocket payments or payments by private long-term care insurance (only in the US did this exceed 0.1 per cent of GDP).[2] Of this amount, home care was seen to account for a small but growing proportion across our countries. Moreover, as emphasised here, because a considerable share of home care in most countries is composed of informal care or privately funded formal care services, its true costs are not reflected in conventional public accounting systems. Thus the real cost to societies of providing home care is significantly higher. Furthermore, because of the demographic and social patterns discussed here, long-term care represents a huge growth area that promises to consume considerably more resources in the coming decades. Not surprisingly, in all of our countries, even New Zealand and the US which lag in many ways, home care has gained increased attention as both a means of controlling the costs of caring for the elderly and on humanistic grounds that ageing in place is preferable to ageing in institutions. Major initiatives in long-term insurance in Japan and Germany are being met with serious initiatives and action across this spectrum of countries.

The provision of home care services is diverse, and this diversity means a greater number and wider range of providers. This requires greater coordination but at the same time makes it more difficult to achieve. Problems of coordination can be exacerbated by a sharp divide between different types of care (for example, health and social care in the UK), the absence of national legislation (as in the case of the US) or a highly decentralised governance structure (as in the case of Sweden). Also it is clear that diversity of provision does not necessarily translate into adequate levels of provision. This gives credence to the more general tenet that in times of cost constraint, diversity of provision frequently coincides with a targeting of services to those in greatest need or those without any other means.

Regardless of the policy trends in the provision and funding of services, home care remains overwhelmingly informal and largely women's work. In comparison to formal home care, informal women's work continues to be cheap and readily available. However, and irrespective of differences among political systems and cultural attitudes towards the role of women, the majority of countries have begun to acknowledge the importance of informal care and the problems it raises for both informal carers and users. These actions take different forms, ranging from the gender blindness of liberal welfare traditions (such as in the US) and challenges to traditional gender-specific expectations in male-dominated, collectivist societies (such as in Japan) to public debates about the relationship between care responsibilities and female labour market participation in welfare societies (the Netherlands and Sweden), the revival of subsidiarity in the context of conservative gender ideas (in Germany), and payments of carers (such as in Estonia, Germany and the Netherlands). What has changed, then, is that the marginality of home care has come into sharper focus and the demographic and social pressure for more extensive and meaningful governance of home care is intensifying.

In our analysis we have uncovered many issues and tensions that underlie this area of governing. These tensions and issues have led to many often highly divergent responses from social and political institutions, sometimes even within a single country. Among the central issues and tensions that accompany home care, we found:

- Family versus public responsibility.
- Institutional versus home care.
- The disconnection between health care and social care and inter-professional rivalries.
- Provision and funding of home care services:
  a. Who sets: government, market, associations?
  b. At what level: national or local?
- Regulations and guidelines:
  a. Who sets: government, market, associations?
  b. At what level: national or local?
- The ill-defined line between formal and informal care.
- Qualifications/training of formal home care workers.
- User choice versus professional dictate.

The remainder of this chapter examines these issues in the light of our analysis in the substantive chapters. What are the varieties of ways in which countries are addressing these tensions? Moreover, if countries tend to cluster around specific types of responses, in what ways does this reflect specific contextual factors in terms of ideas and institutions? It then summarises our findings in terms regarding patterns of convergence and any persistent systematic divergence in governing approaches and policies.

Formal Care Services

The multiple divisions underpinning home care shape the governance of formal care services. Across our countries, the governance of formal care services through funding, delivery and rules is characterised by fragmentation. Variations exist relating to the degree and the type of fragmentation, and the two are closely related. Moreover, the types of fragmentation mirror divisions between public and private provision, between levels of government, as well as between health and social care services. Public provision, integration of health and social care services, and integration of the different levels of governing are all conducive to integrated governing through delivery.

In Chapter 4, we examined the predominant types of funding, delivery and rules relating to formal care giving, and found considerable variation in all areas. Home care clearly exemplifies the tension between health and social care services, and demonstrates the need for coordination and integration of these services. There remain substantial divisions between health and social care services even within specific countries, despite some considerable efforts to integrate such services for the elderly. At present only in Germany, the Netherlands and Sweden is the delivery of health and social services fully integrated. In all other countries, the predominant type of provider varies between these service areas or, in the case of the US and Japan, is a mix of public and private providers.

Often the difference between countries is one of degree, with even those with predominantly public provision revealing a mix of provider types for home care. In like manner, the funding of formal home care can vary not only by country but also between the health and social care components in the same country. Except for social care in the US, however, our countries are evenly split between using taxes and social insurance as the principal funding source. The specific divisions in provision and funding are related to the specific organisation of formal care services, and as such the different types of fragmentation closely mirror the context of governing. Gender cultures and care regimes offer more or less favourable conditions for public provision. Moreover, the relative cohesion (and partly centralisation) of political power facilitates more or less strong integration between different levels of governing.

In summary, formal care is an area of governance that highlights the importance of the divisions between the public and private areas and between national and local levels. It also demonstrates the importance of the characteristics of gender cultures and care regimes for understanding the relative strength of public–private divisions and the consequence of the characteristics of political power over care for understanding the relative strength of national–local divisions.

Informal Care Provision

While formal care is an established area on the policy agenda in our countries, Chapter 5 demonstrated that the issue of informal care givers is quite recent and considerably less settled. Despite this newness, our analysis demonstrates that all countries recognise the mounting problems of informal care and are taking action though often in divergent ways. This variation in strategies is not surprising because the process of change and the newly established mode of delivery, funding and rules have been shaped by ideas and institutions characteristic of different home care approaches. At the base of these developments are the tensions between family and public responsibility of care provision as well as the integration of new actors into the public agenda, particularly care-giver associations, women's groups, unions and user groups.

Across our countries there are two basic modes of inclusion of informal care. The first is a support strategy based on services and the second is a support strategy based on cash benefits. In turn, these two basic strategies can be tied to different ideas that underlie them. Countries oriented towards service provision are generally linked either to ideas of universalism and targeting or to means testing, while the countries oriented towards the cash transfer strategy tend to place more emphasis on family values and responsibilities.

Moreover, as the inclusion of informal care delivery in the overall provision of home care has emerged, the boundary between formal and informal care has become an area of conflict that necessitates innovative forms of cooperation among many institutions. This shift in care regime strategy to support a more integrated notion of home care has resulted in a new symmetry between cash transfers and the provision of in-kind services. This is important because the basic orientation towards a support strategy of services and a support strategy of cash benefits determines the mode of funding, provision and rules related to the integration of informal care provision embedded in different care regimes. Thus New Zealand and the US, with their history of state responsibility only to the needy, have resisted economic support for informal carers, while in the UK the provision of formal care services is the dominant strategy for supporting home care, though only applicants on a low income receive publicly financed social care. Germany, Italy and Estonia, while emphasising family responsibility and care within the family framework, have opted to provide economic support of informal care provision as the principal strategy. In contrast, Japan, Sweden and the Netherlands represent three disparate cultures but they all have care regimes that accept a public responsibility of social care provision for the elderly, primarily through support services.

Since women represent the large majority of informal care givers in all nine of our countries, one cannot ignore the importance of gender cultures and care regimes. Across these countries there are expanding public debates about the relationship between care-giving responsibilities and female labour market participation. Furthermore, these issues are certain to become more important in the future. Although our study did not find ideas on care responsibility inextricably linked with ideas on gender equality related to labour market participation, it is clear that informal care even in the most progressive of our countries continues to be undervalued. This is one area, then, where the tensions might reflect a current weakness of female actors that in the future could be surmounted in part by new coalitions among women's groups and carer groups dominated by female carers.

Formal Care Workers: Redefining Boundaries

As demonstrated in Chapter 6, there has been considerable action in our countries regarding the status of formal care workers for the elderly. First, in some countries the traditional split between professional health care and social care workers has been reduced by efforts to certify care givers. Issues have been raised surrounding the form of such credentials and certification and whether they should be primarily national or local. The formalisation of care arrangements highlights the salient double boundary relative to care workers, that between different levels of training and between formal and informal care work. This tension is the focus of governing and makes for conflicting pressures of reskilling and deskilling. Second, there have been pressures to unionise or otherwise organise care workers. Tensions between professionally trained workers and untrained casual workers are especially common in the more market-driven systems where collective action is minimised.

Our countries are characterised by a number of variations in terms of the relative standing of care workers as trained and paid employees. The relative differentiation of the occupational structure, together with the relative level of qualification, characterises care workers as providers (with the extremes of the prevalence of personal care assistants and a relatively well-qualified workforce). Moreover, the comparative strength of collective agreements is vital for care workers as employees (with complex variations) while the relative importance of different types of rules characterises the regulation of care workers (where hierarchy, also in a variety of hybrids, is prevalent). The variations across our countries reflect a range of contextual factors, including the relative emphasis on formal care services as underpinned by specific gender cultures and care regimes, the specific features of the organisation of formal care services in terms of the health/social care and public/private divide, and country-specific historical developments. In combination these factors offer more or less favourable conditions for the occupational development of care workers as trained and paid employees.

At the practice level there have also been many contemporary initiatives to regulate the training and qualification of formal care workers, although they vary widely in terms of types of workers covered, the extent to which they are uniform nationally, and the respective roles of the state, the market, professional self-regulatory bodies, provider organisations or trade unions in implementing them. Likewise, regulation of occupational territory (either directly or indirectly) varies widely, ranging from national legislation, to local providers, to professional associations, to micro-level decisions by individual care receivers and/or their families. Despite these efforts there continues to be a wide disparity in training levels, and in most of our countries a large proportion of care workers, particularly in the non-health sector, have little or no training or formal qualifications. Although collective agreements in the regulation of salaries are commonplace in all countries except New Zealand and the US, where individual agreements predominate, home care workers at best tend to have relatively lower wages than other health or social service workers, and in some countries on average are barely paid above the minimum wage, often with few benefits. Furthermore, a large proportion of home carers work part time.

In summary, the standing of formal care givers is an area of governance that illustrates the centrality of the boundary between the private and the public, even in relation to an area of governance that is very much related to the public sphere. It also highlights the centrality of the state in relation to the regulation of paid care work, largely irrespective of variations in relation to contextual factors.

Changing Concepts of Home Care Users

In Chapter 7, we focused on three dimensions of user choice in home care: choice among service providers; choice related to content of care provision; and choice between formal and informal care. We found that home care reflects the changing conceptions in the role of users throughout social care provision, and starkly raises the question whether conventional forms of care provision are capable of responding to the escalating diversity of user needs and demands among the elderly. Individual empowerment, social rights and user choice are common catchwords that counter the dominance/dependence patterns of previously entrenched bureaucratic approaches. Across our countries, the introduction of market principles related to the ideas of user choice and competition between providers has become a dominant feature, although variations continue to exist due to the care regime (emphasising public, market and subsidiarity) and the levels of state activities (national/local/regional) involved in decision and implementation. This move towards more consumerist and reconstituted human service approaches based on a mutual bond between provider and an informed user, necessitates a more resourceful relationship among the state, market and family activities.

Investigations into the role of home care users have revealed the difficulties facing many elderly users to act as rational consumers and to take advantage of the different care offerings and opportunities of choice. Against this background, our countries have introduced a variety of measures designed to enable care users to make a more informed choice. Characteristically important for the diverse country approaches is the interplay of regulations on the national and local levels and the type of actors involved.

Social or citizenship rights to care are strongly related to the issue of equal access to care provision. Across our countries, the state is actively redefining social rights and the role of the market, which is decisive for the policies and their realisation. Variation between countries is related to the quality of social rights (public, private responsibility) and linked institutions which are visible in the mode of funding, delivery and rules. Furthermore, variations can be found with regard to the introduction of new state regulations (weak or strict) and the interaction of different state levels.

Defined rules on eligibility and assessment procedures are aimed at guaranteeing equal access to care provision for different user groups. Despite disparities, in all our countries eligibility criteria and assessment procedures have been or are in the process of being established in the context of a diverse interplay of national and local regulations. The tension between the introduction of market mechanisms on the one hand and the ongoing public responsibility and funding of care services on the other has supported the introduction of measures for quality assurance. In all countries the national level is involved in quality assurance regulations with, however, considerable differences in the form of regulations and the level of discretion given to the local levels.

The countries vary with regard to the debates and the availability of these measures. Moreover, the degree to which the various levels are involved in decision making and implementation influence the availability of the measures, for example, the levels of state activities and type of care regime are related. In particular, the care regimes with the idea of public or private responsibility related to modes of care provision, funding and rules, and the interplay of different levels of policy making as well as the integration of new actors (for example, care givers and disabled people's groups and coalitions) seem to determine the speed of change. The development is mainly underpinned with a gender-neutral definition of the users, since the dissimilar societal situations of men and women are rarely considered in the policies and female actors are infrequently involved.

CONVERGENCE OR DIVERGENCE OF HOME CARE GOVERNANCE?

The thematic summary of the governance of home care above reveals the interlocking co-existence of different logics of governance, although the logic of the state dominates. This is interesting, considering that home care is a relatively new area of the welfare *state* and also an area of governance that has traditionally been dominated by the logic of the family and the logic of associations. The relative importance of the logic of the state across our countries also raises questions about the relative importance of convergence and divergence in the governance of home care.

Cross-national demographic and social forces are seen by some observers as reinforcing the *convergence theory*, which holds that as countries industrialise they tend to converge towards the same policy mix (Bennett, 1991). As introduced in Chapter 1, the convergence theory suggests that home care policy across disparate country environments will tend to become more similar over time because similar problems make for similar solutions. Ultimately there are only a limited number of policy instruments available to address a particular policy problem, thus suggesting that function rather than politics informed by historical legacy or culture shapes policy. As Gibson and Means (2000) argue, policy levers are limited and there are simply relatively few 'good ideas' around to solve a specific problem. Convergence is further bolstered by globalisation and by the development of international forums such as the Organisation for Economic Cooperation and Development, the World Health Organisation and the European Union, which provide the grounding for what Harrison et al. (2002) refer to as 'ideational convergence'. These common driving forces, then, suggest a convergence in relation to the framing of policy problems and the intellectual foundations of policy solutions.

In contrast, critics of convergence theories contend that they oversimplify the process of development and underestimate significant divergence across countries (Guillén, 2001). Convergence erroneously downplays the importance of country-specific factors other than economic development, and most studies that find evidence of convergence do not find it applicable across the board, thus allowing for divergence in other areas. Moreover, convergence theory often relies on diffuse variations of 'soft determinism' (Field, 1999), largely based on the assumption that comparable conditions produce comparable problems which result in comparable policies (see Jacobs, 1998).

In his analysis of competing claims about policy convergence and the relative importance of social embeddedness, Saltman (1997) introduces a three-part framework that distinguishes among convergence at the social, political and technical levels. The aspects of policy convergence at the social level include the dominant values and norms of society and its history. The political level in contrast centres on the institutional aspects of convergence such as the structure of the political system, the degree of solidarity versus equity, and the importance of planning versus the market. Finally, the technical/mechanical level includes more instrumental aspects of policy convergence, among them the state of scientific medicine, institutional management and provider payment mechanisms. In his policy analysis, Bennett (1991; similarly Pollitt, 2002) elucidates the concept by distinguishing among convergence in policy goals, policy content and instruments, that is: policy convergence in relation to the intent to deal with common policy problems; in relation to the formal manifestations of government policy; and in relation to the institutional tools to administer policy. Although not rigorously distinct in analytical terms, the three categories nevertheless introduce a dynamic element into the analysis of policy convergence.

One question here, then, is whether the evidence from our nine countries points towards convergence in home care or continued divergence. We suggest that because home care deals with less-standardised, more-personalised services often at the local level, even forces of convergence that might be apparent at national levels are likely to be marginalised or less consistent than in more recognised policy areas. While there has been convergence at the ideational level over the need to address home care as an issue, our findings are mixed in relation to convergence over the framing of home care as a policy problem. At this stage, the wide divergence of home care strategies and priorities across our countries precludes a verdict of policy convergence. Using Saltman's (1997) categorisation scheme, we found no consistent policy convergence at the social, political or technical levels. Although, as illustrated by the summaries of chapters above, we did find clusters of countries that had taken similar routes as to provision, funding or regulation of home care, they were not consistent across all three areas at times even within countries, and they also vary between different substantive areas of governance.

In short, our comparative analysis of the governance of home care tells a story of divergence and of the continued importance of differences across countries. In turn, this raises the question how such differences can be explained. Our analysis suggests that care regimes as social institutions are a central element of the country-specific context that shapes governing arrangements, although not always in a very systematic way. The analysis also points to the importance of political institutions and especially the dynamics between different levels of government. The fragmentation between levels often limits the scope of governing arrangements, whereas the cohesion between levels can offer an important lever for governance. Ideas in the form of gender cultures have an important impact on governing arrangements, although the degree of directness of such influence varies between areas of governance and between countries.

However, the analysis also demonstrates that the explanations of difference are not always consistent, but instead explanations vary between individual governing mechanisms and at times even within countries as well as between different substantive areas of governing. We found systematic variations in some respects but persistent contextually embedded variations (that is, specificities that can be explained based on country-specific constellation of factors) in many other respects. For example, in the case of the governance of care workers in Estonia, the institutional tensions between a care regime that builds on family on the one hand and high as well as mostly full-time female employment on the other, alone cannot explain the high level of training. Instead, the transformation from communism has provided an important lever for change. This raises the question why explanations of differences do not always hold across mechanisms and areas of governance and across countries.

For example, broader cultural differences among our countries are reflected in home care governance. Countries such as Germany, the Netherlands, Japan, Estonia and Italy, with communitarian traditions based either in the family or other groupings, have designed various mechanisms to ensure the interests of the various communities involved with home care. In contrast, countries with egalitarian cultures such as New Zealand, Sweden and the UK place emphasis on the entitlement to a range of home care services and on a societal commitment to provide such care on those grounds, though in the case of New Zealand and the UK these services are often means tested. Finally, the US with its individualistic orientation elevates individual rights above the welfare of the community and largely has viewed home care as an individual or private responsibility. Moreover, the different cultural frameworks of home care are also highly gendered with communitarian and individualistic frameworks heavily relying on unpaid female labour of love (by design and default, respectively), whereas the egalitarian framework partly recognises the provision of care as a public responsibility.

Yet our analysis demonstrates that the relationship between ideas about gender culture and home care governance is complicated. Although home care is a highly gendered area of governance, ideas about gender culture do not necessarily always feature explicitly in the development of policies. Analytically this raises questions about the specific meaning of gender in relation to governing home care. Here we suggest distinguishing between three types of influence: first, implicit influence whereby salient ideas about gender culture inform the development of policies; second, explicit influence whereby ideas about gender culture openly feature in public debates about policy development; and third, agency-based influence whereby ideas about gender culture influence policy development by virtue of the inclusion of female collective actors. Our analysis suggests that the first type of influence is most important, although in many of our countries the increasing female labour market participation and the corresponding changes in gender culture are openly discussed (the second type of influence). This often serves as an incentive for the development of new policies. In contrast, the involvement of female collective actors in processes of policy development (the third type of influence) is even rarer, and among our countries only in Japan and Sweden did we find an increase in the influence of such actors. In addition, the rising impact of carer groups dominated by female carers since the 1990s offers opportunities for new coalitions between female actors and the formation of a new type of gendered influence on policy development.

Further, while cultural differences remain important determinants of home care governance, however, our analysis does indicate a tension between these traditional cultural settings and the realities all countries face in devising workable strategies to deal with rapidly ageing populations, mounting economic constraints on both governments and families, and social changes that are significantly reducing the capacity of families to take care of their own. One tension is manifest in the move of most countries towards inclusion of market approaches, even those countries that until now have resisted markets in other areas. Similarly, the tension between family and social responsibility most starkly illustrated in Japan is present across these countries, and leads to apparent discrepancies, for example, in the US where the motivation for shifting emphasis from the residential to the home care setting is primarily an effort to contain burgeoning health care and institutional costs.

The inconsistencies in the applicability of contextual factors as explanatory factors to some extent might simply be a function of the nature of comparison and of the attempt here to combine an analysis of institutions and cultural approaches since institutional approaches have an inherent promise about systematic variations while cultural approaches, suggest understanding variations only on the basis of in-depth country-specific cases. Furthermore, Anttonen et al. (2003b) suggest that the paucity of systematic variations in home care governance has to do with the plasticity of care, especially the interchangeability between formal and informal care and the associated importance of dynamics. Culture understood as values and expectations underpinning home care arrangements therefore may be a more important reference point and, by extension, a framework for comparison. Another explanation, however, could be that the variations relating to the contextual factors as the independent variable are not very strong. In relation to ideas, for example, our countries clustered around variants of the female carer model. It is significant here that we principally found disparities at the extremes, for example, Sweden versus Italy. Similarly, the political power over home care is relatively cohesive in most countries, and apart from outliers such as Italy and the US, the divergence is one of variations in degree not direction.

CONCLUSIONS

From the discussion above it is clear that the analytical framework presented in Chapter 1 does not apply uniformly across our countries. Although the context of the countries is very similar notwithstanding the area of governance we are discussing, contextual factors come into play very differently across our four areas of governance. For example, in relation to care users from different perspectives on development, dissimilar features of the care regime are emphasised, resulting in different assignments of the countries in each of the three sections. Moreover, in relation to some areas of governance, additional contextual factors come into play. In the case of care workers, for instance, the regulation of salaries has to be understood against the background of the type of labour relations typical of a country. This complexity in particular applies to Chapters 6 and 7 on care workers and users that do not neatly fall into either formal care services or informal care.

In conclusion, home care is a relatively new and unsettled area on the political agendas of most of these countries but three sets of factors – demographic, social and economic – have combined to create a dynamic and fluid environment for the governance of home care. Perhaps because of this recency, home care is full of contradictions. While it is a vital need across all countries, governance is varied and diverse in detail. Moreover, while home care is hardly discernible in international statistics on spending, it is crucial to the health and well-being of an increasing number of people. Home care funding and provision is frequently fragmented and in some cases lacking order, yet it is of increasing importance on the policy agenda of these countries.

Home care governance has become a salient matter of public concern in all of our countries as well as a defining issue in the reorganisation of social services and the interplay of the public and private sectors. Demographic and social forces, along with moves towards more consumerist approaches in combination, are leading to essential changes in the delivery, funding and governance of care for the elderly. These changes in turn necessitate new cooperative instruments that amalgamate the strengths of the until-recently competing logics of the state, the market and the family. To a varying degree, home care governance has become a dynamic and lively issue in all these countries and has brought many new actors into the public arena. It also has generated many tensions that will serve as the basis for vigorous debate and action in the coming decades as societies cope with the broadened demand for more user-friendly and diverse packages of services designed to allow the elderly to age in place. Clearly the resolution of these tensions will require enlightened thinking by a new breed of public and private leaders who can mould the disparate needs and demands of a wide variety of parties into workable and sustainable home care schemes.

NOTES

1. We realise that our analysis by its breadth is relatively superficial as to each country and that a full analysis of each country is needed to be authoritative.
2. One problem we found in our comparative analysis was the difficulty of obtaining accurate data on home care for most countries, much less to provide reliable comparative data. Part of this problem stems from the disparate nature of home care discussed above, and part because it is a relatively new policy area in most countries. Moreover, often the public expenditures are included in residential care under the rubric of long-term care, thus blurring the actual amount going to home care.

Bibliography

Aimar, Bruno, Enzo Bozza, Maria Grazia Breda, Emanuela Buffa, Donata Micucci, Mauro Perino and Francesco Santanera (2004), 'La pilatesca risposta della Presidenza della Repubblica alle preoccupanti emergenze segnalate', *Prospettive Assistenziali*, **146**, 25–7.

Alber, Jens (1995), 'A framework for the comparative study of social services', *Journal of European Social Policy*, **5** (2), 131–50.

Alber, Jens and Martin Schölkopf (1999), *Seniorenpolitik: Die Soziale Lage älterer Menschen in Deutschland und Europa*, Amsterdam: Fakultas Verlag.

Alber, Jens and Ulrich Köhler (2004), *Health and Care in an Enlarged Europe*, European Foundation for the Improvement Working Conditions, Official Publications of the European Communities, Luxembourg, www.fr.eurofound.eu.int/publications/files/EF03107EN.pdf, 10 July 2006.

American Society on Aging (2006), *Profile of Informal and Family Caregivers*, www.asaging.org/pew/feinberg/feinberg-profile.html, 5 February 2007.

Andall, J. (2000), *Gender, Migration and Domestic Service: The Politics of Black Women in Italy*, Aldershot: Ashgate.

Anttonen, Anneli and Jorma Sipilä (1996), 'European social care services: is it possible to identify models?', *Journal of European Social Policy*, **6** (2), 87–100.

Anttonen, Anneli, John Baldock and Jorma Sipilä (eds) (2003a), *The Young, the Old and the State: Social Care Systems in Five Industrial Nations*, Cheltenham, UK and Northampton, MA, USA: Edward Elgar.

Anttonen, Anneli, Jorma Sipilä and John Baldock (2003b), 'Patterns of social care in five industrial societies: explaining diversity', in Anneli Anttonen, John Baldock and Jorma Sipilä (eds), *The Young, the Old and the State: Social Care Systems in Five Industrial Nations*, Cheltenham, UK and Northampton, MA, USA: Edward Elgar, pp. 167–97.

Arai, Yumiko and Keigo Kumamoto (2004), 'Caregiver burden not "worse" after new public long-term care (LTC) insurance scheme took over in Japan', *International Journal of Geriatric Psychiatry*, **19**, 1205–6.

Ashton, Toni (2000), 'New Zealand: long-term care in a decade of change', *Health Affairs*, **19** (3), 72–81.

Baggot, Rob, Judith Allsop and Kathryn Jones (2005), *Speaking for Patients and Carers: Health Consumer Groups and the Policy Process*, Basingstoke: Palgrave Macmillan.

Baldock, John (1998), 'Old age, consumerism and the social care market', in Edward Brundson, Hartley Dean and Roberta Woods (eds), *Social Policy Review 10*, Canterbury: Social Policy Association, pp. 165–82.

Baldock, John (2003), 'Social care in the United Kingdom: a pattern of discretionary social administration', in Anneli Anttonen, John Baldock and Jorma Sipilä (eds), *The Young, the Old and the State: Social Care Systems in Five Industrial Nations*, Cheltenham, UK and Northampton, MA, USA: Edward Elgar, pp. 109–41.

Bamber, Greg, Russell D. Lansbury and Nick Wailes (eds) (2004), *International and Comparative Employment Relations. Globalisation and the Developed Market Economies*, London: Sage.

Barnes, Marian (2001), 'From private carer to public actor: the carers' movement in England', in Mary Daly (ed.), *Care Work: The Quest for Security*, Geneva: International Labour Organization, pp. 195–209.

Barnes, Marian, Steve Harrison, Maggie Mort, Polly Shardlow and Gerald Wistow (1999), 'The new management of community care: user groups, citizenship and co-production', in Gerry Stoker (ed.), *The New Management of British Local Governance*, Basingstoke: Palgrave, pp. 112–27.

Baumgartner, Frank B. and Bryan Jones (1991), 'Agenda setting and policy subsystems', *Journal of Politics*, **53** (4), 1045–74.

Beck Jørgensen, Torben and Karsten Vrangbæk (2004), *Det Offentlige Styringsunivers. Fra Government til Governance?* Aarhus: Aarhus Universitetsforlag.

Bennett, Colin J. (1991), 'What is policy convergence and what causes it?', *British Journal of Political Science*, **21** (2), 215–33.

Benoit, Cecilia and Alena Heitlinger (1998), 'Women's health care work in comparative perspective: Canada, Sweden and Czechoslovakia/Czech Republic as case examples', *Social Science and Medicine*, **47** (8), 1101–11.

Bettio, Francesca and Janneke Plantenga (2004), 'Comparing care regimes in Europe', *Feminist Economics*, **10** (1), 85–113.

Björkman, James Warner and Kieke G.H. Okma (1997), 'Restructuring health care systems in the Netherlands: the institutional heritage of Dutch health policy reforms', in Christa Altenstetter and James Warner Björkman (eds), *Health Policy Reform, National Variations and Globalization*, Basingstoke: Macmillan, pp. 79–108.

Blackman, Tim, Sally Brodhurst and Janet Convery (eds) (2001), *Social Care and Social Exclusion: A Comparative Study of Older People's Care in Europe*, Basingstoke: Palgrave.

Bleich, Erik (2002), 'Integrating ideas into policy-making analysis: frames and race policies in Britain and France', *Comparative Political Studies*, **35** (9), 1054–76.

Blinkert, Baldo and Thomas Klie (1999), *Pflege im sozialen Wandel: Studie Zur Situation Häuslich Versorgter Pflegebedürftiger*, Hannover: Vincentz-Verlag.

Bonoli, Giuliano (2005), 'The politics of the new social policies: providing coverage against new social risks in mature welfare states', *Policy and Politics*, **33** (3), 431–49.

Boom, Hannerieke van der (forthcoming), *A Comparative, Contextual Perspective on Home Nursing in Europe: An Institutional Analysis of the Relations between Home Nursing, Home Help and Informal Care in Denmark, France, Germany and The Netherlands*, Maastricht: Department of Health Care Studies, Maastricht University.

Boom, Hannerieke van der, Fred Stevens and Hans Philipsen (2004), 'Caring for frail elderly and chronically ill people: the triad of home nursing, home help and family care in Denmark, the Netherlands and France', Paper presented at the 4th Interim Conference of the Research Committee 52 'Sociology of Professional Groups' of the International Sociological Association, Versailles, France, 22–24 September.

Braun, Dietmar (1999), 'Interests and ideas? An overview of ideational concepts in public policy research', in Dietmar Braun and Andreas Busch (eds), *Public Policy and Political Ideas*, Cheltenham, UK and Northampton, MA, USA: Edward Elgar, pp. 11–29.

Briskin, Linda (1999), 'Mapping women's organizing in Sweden and Canada: some thematic considerations', in Linda Briskin and Mona Eliasson (eds), *Women's Organizing and Public Policy in Canada and Sweden*, Montreal and Kingston: McGill-Queen's University Press, pp. 3–50.

Brodhurst, Sally and Caroline Glendinning (2001), 'The United Kingdom', in Tim Blackman, Sally Brodhurst and Janet Convery (eds), *Social Care and Social Exclusion: A Comparative Study of Older People's Care in Europe*, Basingstoke: Palgrave, pp. 68–82.

Brodin, Helene (2005), 'Does anybody care? Public and private responsibilities in Swedish eldercare 1940–2000', Doctoral thesis, University of Umeå, Umeå, Sweden.

Bundesministerium für Gesundheit (2004), *Dritter Bericht zur Entwicklung der Pflegeversicherung*, Berlin: Bundesministerium für Gesundheit.

Burau, Viola (2005), 'Comparing professions through actor-centred governance: community nursing in Britain and Germany', *Sociology of Health and Illness*, **27** (1), 114–37.

Burau, Viola and Teppo Kröger (2004), 'Towards local comparisons of community care governance: exploring the relationship between policy and politics', *Social Policy and Administration*, **38** (7), 793–810.

Busch, Andreas and Dietmar Braun (1999), 'Introduction', in Dietmar Braun and Andreas Busch (eds), *Public Policy and Political Ideas*, Cheltenham, UK and Northampton, MA, USA: Edward Elgar, pp. 1–7.

Cameron, Clare and Peter Moss (2001), *Mapping Care Services and the Care Workforce, National Report, United Kingdom* (Work Package 3 of 'Care work in Europe. Current understanding and future directions'), London: Institute for Education, University of London.

Cameron, Claire and Peter Moss (2002a), *Surveying Demand, Supply and Use of Care, National Report, United Kingdom* (Work Package 4 of 'Care work in Europe. Current understandings and future directions'), London: Institute for Education, University of London.

Cameron, Clare and Peter Moss (2002b), *Literature Review Since 1990 on Job Satisfaction, Quality and Aspects of Diversity in the Care Workforce, National Report, United Kingdom* (Work Package 5 of 'Care work in Europe. Current understanding and future directions'), London: Institute for Education, University of London.

Campbell, John Creighton and Naoki Ikegami (2003), 'Japan's radical reform of long-term care', *Social Policy and Administration*, **37** (1), 21–34.

Campbell, Andrea Louise and Kimberly J. Morgan (2005), 'Federalism and the politics of old-age care in Germany and the United States', *Comparative Political Studies*, **38** (8), 1–28, 997–1014.

Caplan, G.A., J.A. Ward, N.J. Brennan, J. Coconis, N. Board and Ann Brown (1999), 'Hospital in the home: a randomised controlled trial', *Medical Journal of Australia*, **170**, 156–60.

Carers UK (2001), 'Carers and Disabled Children Act 2000. Policy and practice guidance. Briefing for carers' groups and carers' organisations', www.carersuk.org/Policyandpractice/PolicyResources/Policybriefings, 17 August 2006.

Carers UK (2005), 'Carers and Disabled Children Act 2000 & Carers (Equal Opportunities) Act 2004. Carers UK's response to the combined draft policy guidance. March 2005', www.carersuk.org/Policyandpractice/PolicyResources/Policybriefings, 17 August 2006.

Carers UK (nd), 'Carers UK success and achievements', www.carersuk.org/Aboutus/AboutCarersUK/CarersUKsuccess, 17 August 2006.

Centers for Medicare and Medicaid Services (2003a), *Medicare and Home Health Care*, Washington, DC: Government Printing Office.

Centers for Medicare and Medicaid Services (2003b), 'Alternatives to Nursing Home Care', www.medicare.gov/Nursing/Alternatives/Other.asp, 5 February 2007.

Centrum Indicatiestelling Zorg (nd), www.ciz.nl/, 5 February 2007.

Charles, Nickie (2000), *Feminism, the State and Social Policy*, Basingstoke: Macmillan.

Clarke, John (nd), 'Consumers, clients or citizens? Politicism policy and practice in the reform of social care', Unpublished manuscript, Milton Keynes: Open University.

Clarke, John, Nick Smith and Elizabeth Vidler (2005), 'Consumerism and the reform of public services: inequalities and instabilities', *Social Policy Review*, **17**, 167–82.

Colombo, A. (2003), 'Razza, genere, classe. Le tre dimensioni del lavoro domestico in Italia', *Polis*, **2**, 317–42.

Convery, Janet and Elisabetta Cioni (2001), 'Italy', in Tim Blackman, Sally Brodhurst and Janet Convery (eds), *Social Care and Social Exclusion: A Comparative Study of Older People's Care in Europe*, Basingstoke: Palgrave, pp. 68–82.

Conway, M. Margaret, David W. Ahern and Gertrude A. Steuernagel (1998), *Women and Public Policy*, Washington, DC: Congressional Quarterly.

Coolen, Jan and Sylvia Weekers (1998), 'Long-term care in the Netherlands: public funding and private provision within a universalistic welfare state', in Caroline Glendinning (ed.), *Rights and Realities: Comparing New Developments in Long-term Care for Older People*, Bristol: Policy Press, pp. 47–66.

Cuellar, A.E. and J.M. Wiener (2000), 'Can social insurance for long term care work? The experience of Germany', *Health Affairs*, **19** (3), 8–39.

Da Roit, B. (2005), 'Convergenze e divergenze nelle politiche sociosanitarie regionali per gli anziani in Lombardia, Emilia-Romagna e Veneto', in Carla Facchini (ed.), *Anziani e sistemi di Welfare. Lombardia, Italia, Europa. Rapporto 2005 Spi-Cgil-Cadef*, Milan: Franco Angeli, pp. 181–230.

Dahlberg, Lena (2005), 'Interaction between voluntary and statutory service provisions: a matter of welfare pluralism, substitution or complementarity?', *Social Policy and Administration*, **39** (7), 740–63.

Dahlerup, Drude (1987), 'Confusing concepts – confusing reality: a theoretical discussion of the patriarchal state', in Anne Showstack Sassoon (ed.), *Women and the State*, London: Hutchinson, pp. 93–127.

Daly, Mary (2000), 'Care policies in Western Europe', in Mary Daly (ed.), *Care Work: The Quest for Security*, Geneva: International Labour Office, pp. 33–56.

Daly, Mary (2002), 'Care as a good for social policy', *Journal of Social Policy*, **31** (2), 251–70.

Daly, Mary (2003), 'Governance and social policy', *Journal of Social Policy*, **32** (1), 113–28.

Daly, Mary and Jane Lewis (1998), 'Introduction: conceptualising social care in the context of welfare state restructuring', in Jane Lewis (ed.), *Gender, Social Care and Welfare State Restructuring in Europe*, Aldershot: Ashgate, pp. 1–24.

Daly, Mary and Jane Lewis (2000), 'The concept of social care and the analysis of contemporary welfare states', *British Journal of Sociology*, **51** (2), 281–98.

Daly, Mary and Katherine Rake (2003), *Gender and the Welfare State: Care, Work and Welfare in Europe and the USA*, Cambridge: Polity Press.

Davey, Judith A. (2002), *Needs Assessment for the Over 65s*, Wellington: New Zealand Institute for Research on Ageing.

Davey, Judith A. and Sally Keeling (2004), 'Combining work and eldercare: a neglected work–life balance issue', in *Labour, Employment and Work in New Zealand*, Wellington: Victoria University Institute for Research on Ageing.

Delevett, Peter (1999), 'Home health care suffers from increased regulations', *The Business Journal*, **16** (42), 28.

Dent, Mike (2003), *Remodelling Hospitals and Health Professions in Europe: Medicine, Nursing and the State*, Basingstoke: Palgrave.

Department of Work and Pensions/National Statistics (2004), *Work and Pensions Statistics 2004*, Newcastle-upon-Tyne: Department of Work and Pensions.

Deutscher Bundestag (2004), *Dritter Bericht über die Entwicklung der Pflegeversicherung*, Drucksache 15/4125, Berlin: Deutscher Bundestag.

DHBNZ (District Health Boards New Zealand) (2004), 'Workforce Action Plan 2004/05 Projects and Development', Unpublished report.

Duff, John (2001), 'Financing to foster community health care: a comparative analysis of Singapore, Europe, North America, and Australia', *Current Sociology*, **49** (3), 135–54.

Edebalk, Per Gunnar and Marianne Svensson (2005), *Kundval för äldre och funktionshindrade i Norden*, TemaNord 2005:507, Köpenhamn: Nordiska Ministerrådet.

Escobedo, Anna, Esther Fernandez, David Moreno and Peter Moss (eds) (2002), *Surveying Demand, Supply and Use of Care: Consolidated Report* (Work Package 4 of 'Care work in Europe. Current understandings and future directions'), Barcelona/London: Fundación CIREM/Institute for Education, University of London.

Esping-Andersen, Gøsta (1990), *The Three Worlds of Welfare Capitalism*, Princeton, NJ: Princeton University Press.

Eto, Mikiko (2001), 'Public involvement in social policy reform: seen from the perspective of Japan's elderly-care insurance scheme', *Journal of Social Policy*, **30** (1), 17–36.

European Commission (2005), *Employment in Europe*, Directorate-General for Employment, Social Affairs and Equal Opportunities, Brussels.

European Foundation for the Improvement of Living and Working Conditions

(2006), *Employment in Social Care*, Dublin: European Foundation for the Improvement of Living and Working Conditions.

European Observatory on Health Care Systems (2001), *Health Care Systems in Transition: Italy*, Copenhagen: European Observatory on Health Care Systems, www.euro.who.int/document/e73096.pdf, 5 February 2007.

European Observatory on Health Systems and Policies (2004), *Health Care Systems in Transition: Netherlands*, Copenhagen: European Observatory on Health Systems and Policies.

Eurostat (1999), '"Profound Consequences" as EU Grows Older', News Release 75/99, 29 July.

Evers, Adalbert and Ivan Svetlik (eds) (1993), *Balancing Pluralism: New Welfare Mixes in Care for the Elderly*, Aldershot: Avebury.

Evers, Adalbert and Helmut Wintersberger (eds) (1990), *Shifts in the Welfare Mix*, Frankfurt am Main: Campus.

Ewijk, Hans van (2002), *Surveying Demand, Supply and Use of Care, National Report, Netherlands* (Work Package 4 of 'Care work in Europe. Current understanding and future directions'), Utrecht: Nederlands Institute for Care and Welfare.

Ewijk, Hans van, Harry Hens and Gery Lammerson (2002), *Mapping Care Service and the Care Workforce, National Report, Netherlands* (Work Package 3 of 'Care work in Europe. Current understandings and future directions'), Utrecht: Nederlands Institute for Care and Welfare.

Exter, André, Herbert Hermans, Milena Dosljak and Reinhard Busse (2004), *Health Care Systems in Transition: Netherlands*, Copenhagen: WHO Regional Office for Europe on behalf of the European Observatory on Health Care Systems.

Family Caregiver Alliance (2006), 'Work and eldercare', www.caregiver.org/caregiver/jsp/content_node.jsp?nodeid=413, 5 February 2007.

Fargion, Valeria (2005), 'From the southern to the northern question: territorial and social policy', in Nicola McEwen and Luis Moreno (eds), *The Territorial Politics of Welfare*, London: Routledge, pp. 127–47.

Federal Statistical Office (2003), *Pflegestatistik 2001*, Bonn, www.destatis.de, 5 February 2007.

Federal Statistical Office (2005a), *Länderbericht Pflegebedürftige*, Bonn, www.destatis.de, 5 February 2007.

Federal Statistical Office (2005b), *Ländervergleich ambulante Pflegedienste*, Bonn, www.destatis.de, 5 February 2007.

Federal Statistical Office (2005c), *Deutschlandergebnisse*, Bonn, www.destatis.de, 5 February 2007.

Federal Statistical Office (2005d), *Leistungen der Pflegeversicherung für Ältere. Unveröffentlichter Bericht*, Bonn.

Feltenius, David (2004), 'En Pluralistisk Maktordning? Om

Pensionärsorganisationerna Politiska Inflyttande', Doctoral thesis, University of Umeå, Umeå, Sweden.

Ferioli, E.A. (2004), 'Pronunce costituzionali sui servizi sociali', *Prospettive Sociali e Sanitarie*, **34** (19), 1–3.

Field, M.G. (1999), 'Comparative health systems and the convergence hypothesis: the dialectics of universalism and particularism', in F.D. Powell and A.F. Wessen (eds), *Health Care Systems in Transition: An International Perspective*, Thousand Oaks, CA: Sage, pp. 35–44.

Finch, Janet (1989), *Family Obligations and Social Change*, London: Polity Press.

Finch, Janet and Dulcie Groves (eds) (1983), *A Labour of Love: Women, Work and Caring*, London: Routledge & Kegan Paul.

Finch, Janet and Jennifer Mason (1991), *Negotiating Family Responsibilities*, London/New York: Tavistock/Routledge.

Finch, Janet and Jennifer Mason (1993), 'Obligations of kinship in contemporary Britain. Is there normative agreement?', *British Journal of Sociology*, **42** (3), 345–67.

Forder, Julien, Martin Knapp, Brian Hardy, Jeremy Kendall, Tihana Matosevic and Patricia Ware (2004), 'Prices, contracts and motivations: institutional arrangements in domiciliary care', *Policy and Politics*, **32** (2), 207–22.

Freeman, Gary P. (1985), 'National styles and policy sectors: explaining structured variation', *Journal of Public Policy*, **5** (4), 467–96.

Freeman, Richard (2000), *The Politics of Health in Europe*, Manchester: Manchester University Press.

Fujiwara, Kyoko, Eri Tsukishima, Akizumi Tsutsumi, Norita Kawakami and Rieko Kishi (2003), 'Interpersonal conflict, social support, and burnout among home care workers in Japan', *Journal of Occupational Health*, **45**, 313–20.

Gerste, Bettina and Isabel Rehbein (1998), *Der Pflegemarkt in Deutschland*, Bonn: Wissenschaftliches Institut der AOK.

Gibson, Diane and Robin Means (2000), 'Policy convergence: restructuring long-term care in Australia and the UK', *Policy and Politics*, **29** (1), 43–58.

Giese, Reinhard and Dieter Wiegel (2000), *Veränderungen durch die Pflegeversicherung in der häuslichen Pflege. Vortrag zur Ringvorlesung Altersforschung in Hamburg*, Arbeitsstelle für Rehabilitations- und Präventionsforschung: Universität Hamburg.

Ginn, Jay and Sara Arber (1999), 'The politics of old age in the UK', in Alan Walker and Gerhard Nægele (eds), *The Politics of Old Age in Europe*, Buckingham: Open University Press, pp. 152–67.

Giullari, Susy and Jane Lewis (2005), 'The adult worker model family, gender equality and care: the search for new policy principles and the possibilities and problems of a capabilities approach', United Nations Research Institute for Social Development, Social Policy and Development Programme, paper number 19, April.

Glendinning, Caroline (1998), 'Health and social care services for frail older people in the UK: changing responsibilities and new developments', in Caroline Glendinning (ed.), *Rights and Realities: Comparing New Developments in Long-term Care for Older People*, Bristol: Policy Press, pp. 11–28.

Gori, Cristiano (ed.) (2002), *Il welfare nascosto. Il mercato privato dell'assistenza in Italia e in Europa*, Rome: Carocci Editore.

Gough, Ritva (1994), 'Från hembiträden till social hemtjänst', in Annika Baude and Cecilia Rundström (eds), *Kvinnans plats i det tidiga välfärdssamhället*, Stockholm: Carlsson, pp. 39–56.

Graham, Hillary (1991), 'The concept of caring in feminist research. The case of domestic service', *Sociology*, **25**, 61–78.

Greiner, Wolfgang and J.-Matthias Graf von der Schulenburg (1997), 'Germany', in Marshall W. Raffel (ed.), *Health Care and Reform in Industrialized Countries*, University Park, PA: Pennsylvania State University Press, pp. 77–104.

Guillén, Mauro F. (2001), *The Limits of Convergence: Globalization and Organizational Change in Argentina, South Korea and Spain*, Princeton, NJ: Princeton University Press.

Gundling, Richard (2000), 'Home health agencies should prepare for prospective payment', *Healthcare Financial Management*, **54** (2), 72, February.

Håkansson, Stefan and Sara Nordling (1997), 'Sweden', in Marshall W. Raffel (ed.), *Health Care and Reform in Industrialized Countries*, University Park, PA: Pennsylvania State University Press, pp. 191–226.

Hall, Peter A. (1993), 'Policy paradigms, social learning, and the state: the case of economic policymaking in Britain', *Comparative Politics*, **25** (3), 275–96.

Hall, Peter A. and Rosemary C.R. Taylor (1996), 'Political science and the three institutionalisms', *Political Studies*, **44** (5), 936–57.

Ham, Chris (ed.) (1997), *Health Care Reform: Learning from International Experience*, Buckingham: Open University Press.

Harrison, Stephen, Michael Moran and Bruce Wood (2002), 'Policy emergence and policy convergence: the case of "scientific-bureaucratic medicine" in the United States and United Kingdom', *British Journal of Politics and International Relations*, **4** (1), 1–24.

Harrop, M. (1992), 'Introduction', in M. Harrop (ed.), *Power and Policy in Liberal Democracies*, Cambridge: Cambridge University Press.

Heidenheimer, Arnold Jospeh, Hugh Heclo and Carolyn Teich Adams (1983),

Comparative Public Policy: The Politics of Social Choice in Europe and America, 2nd edn, Basingstoke: Macmillan.

Henriksson, Lea, Sirpa Wrede and Viola Burau (2006), 'Understanding professional projects in welfare service work: revival of old professionalism?', *Gender, Work and Organization*, **13** (2), 174–92.

Hernes, Helga Maria (1984), 'Women and the welfare state: the transition from private to public dependence', in Harriet Holter (ed.), *Patriarchy in a Welfare Society*, Oslo: Universitetsförlaget, pp. 26–45.

Hernes, Helga Maria (1987a), *Welfare State and Women Power*, Oslo: Norwegian University Press.

Hernes, Helga Maria (1987b), 'Women and the welfare state: the transition from private to public dependence', in Anne Showstack Sassoon (ed.), *Women and the State*, London: Hutchinson, pp. 72–92.

Heywood, Andrew (1997), *Politics*, Basingstoke: Macmillan.

Hillmann, Felicitas (2005), 'Migrants' care work in private households, or the strength of bilocal and transnational ties as a last(ing) resource in global migration', in Birgit Pfau-Effinger and Birgit Geissler (eds), *Care and Social Integration in European Societies*, Bristol: Policy Press, pp. 93–112.

Hirdman, Yvonne (1990), *Genussystemet*, in SOU, *Demokrati och Makt i Sverige, Maktutredningens huvudrapport*, Stockholm: Allmänna Förlag, pp. 73–116.

Hjalmarson, Ingrid (2006), *Man söker inte hjälp i onödan*, Rapporter Stiftelsen Stockholms läns Äldrecentrum (Stockholm Gerontology Research Center), 2006:1.

Hochschild, Arlie Russel (1995), 'The culture of politics: traditional, post-modern, cold-modern and warm-modern ideals of care', *Social Politics*, **2** (3), 333–46.

Hochschild, Arlie Russel (2000), 'The nanny chain', *The American Prospect*, **11** (4), 32–6.

Hojlund, Holger (2005), 'At give de ældre røst – Tre brugerorienterede tillgange till utviklingen i ældresektoren', in Marta Szebehely (ed.), *Äldreomsorgsforskning i Norden*, En kunskapsöversikt, Tema Nord 2005:508, Köpenhamn: Nordiska Ministerrådet, pp. 113–42.

Hondagneu-Sotelo, Pierrette (2000), 'The international division of caring and cleaning work', in Madonna Harrington Meyer (ed.), *Care Work: Gender, Class and the Welfare State*, London and New York: Routledge, pp. 149–62.

Howlett, Michael and M. Ramesh (2003), *Studying Public Policy: Policy Cycles and Policy Subsystems*, 2nd edn, Oxford: Oxford University Press.

Hrebenar, Ronald J., Akira Nakainura and Akio Nakamura (1998), 'Lobby regulation in the Japanese diet', *Parliamentary Affairs*, **51**, 551–8.

Hudson, Brian and Melanie Henwood (2002), 'The NHS and social care: the final countdown?' *Policy and Politics*, **30** (2), 153–66.

Hutton, Jack B.F. (1996), 'Home care in Italy', in Jack B.F. Hutton and Ada Kerkstra (eds), *Home Care in Europe: Country-specific Guide to its Organization and Financing*, Aldershot: Ashgate, pp. 184–203.

Igl, Gerhard and Felix Welti (1999), 'Öffentlich-rechtliche Grundlagen für die Entwicklung vorbehaltener Aufgabenbereiche im Berufsfeld Pflege', *Vierteljahresschrift für Sozialrecht*, **1**, 21–55.

Ikegami, N. (1992), 'Japan: maintaining equity through regulated fees', *Journal of Health Politics, Policy and Law*, **17** (4), 689–713.

Ikegami, Naoki and John Creighton Campbell (2002), 'Choices, policy logics and problems in the design of long-term care systems', *Social Policy and Administration*, **36** (7), 719–34.

Ikegami, Naoki, Keita Yamauchi and Yukari Yamada (2003), 'The long term care insurance law in Japan: impact on institutional care facilities', *International Journal of Geriatric Psychiatry*, **18**, 217–21.

Immergut, Ellen M. (1992), *Health Politics: Interests and Institutions in Western Europe*, Cambridge: Cambridge University Press.

International Reform Monitor (nd), *Country Information: Italy. Health Care and Long Term Care*, www.reformmonitor.org/index.php3?mode=status, 23 August 2006.

Izuhara, Misa (2003), 'Social inequality under a new social contract: long-term care in Japan', *Social Policy and Administration*, **37** (4), 395–410.

Jacobs, Alan (1998), 'Seeing difference: market health reform in Europe', *Journal of Health Politics, Policy and Law*, **23** (1), 1–33.

Jacobzone, Stephane (1999), 'Ageing and care for frail elderly persons: an overview of international perspectives', Labour Market and Social Policy Occasional Papers 38, Paris: OECD.

Jamieson, Anne (1996), 'Issues in home care services', Caring for Frail Elderly People: Policies in Evolution, Social Policy Studies 19, Paris: OECD.

Japan Ministry of Health, Labour and Welfare (1999), *Annual Report on Health and Welfare: Social Security and National Life*, Tokyo: Ministry of Health, Labour and Welfare.

Japan Ministry of Health, Labour and Welfare (2002), *Long-term Care Insurance in Japan*, Tokyo: Ministry of Health, Labour and Welfare.

Japan Ministry of Health, Labour and Welfare (2004a), 'Negotiating family support? The "generational contract" between long-term care and inheritance', *International Social Policy*, **33** (4), 649–65.

Japan Ministry of Health, Labour and Welfare (2004b), *Direction of Health and Welfare Policies for the Elderly over the Next 5 Years*, Tokyo: Ministry of Health, Labour and Welfare.

Jenson, Jane and Stephane Jacobzone (2000), 'Care allowances for the frail elderly and their impact on women care-givers', Labour Market and Social Policy Occasional Papers 41, Paris: OECD.

Jessop, Bob (1999), 'The changing governance of welfare: recent trends in its primary functions, scale, and modes of coordination', *Social Policy and Administration*, **22** (4), 348–39.

Johansson, Lennart (2004), 'National Background Report for Sweden', EU-Project EUROFAMCARE, Hamburg, www.uke.uni-hamburg.de/EUROFAMCARE, 5 February 2007.

Johansson, Sunne (1997), 'Hälsoprofessioner i välfärdsstatens omvandling', in Elisabeth Sundin (ed.), *Om makt och kön*, Stockholm: Arbetsmarknadsdepartement, pp. 69–102.

Johansson, Stina and Peter Moss (2004), *Work with Elderly People. A Case Study of Sweden, Spain and England with Additional Material from Hungary. Consolidated Report* (Work Package 9 of 'Care work in Europe: Current understanding and future directions'), London: Institute for Education, University of London.

Johnson, M. and L. Cullen (2000), 'Solidarity put to the test. Health and social care in the UK', *Journal of International Social Welfare*, **9**, 228–37.

Johnson, Norman (2001), 'The personal social services', in Stephen P. Savage and Rob Atkinson (eds), *Public Policy under Blair*, Basingstoke: Palgrave, pp. 174–61.

Jordan, Grant and William A. Maloney (1997), 'Accounting for subgovernments. Explaining the persistence of policy communities', *Administration and Society*, **29** (5), 557–83.

Kadushin, Goldie (2004), 'Home health care utilization: a review of the research for social work', *Health and Social Work*, **29** (3), 219–32.

Karlsson, Martin, Les Mayhew, Robert Plumb and Ben Rickayzen (2004), 'An international comparison of long-term care arrangements', *Actuarial Research Centre*, (156), 1–131.

Kaupuza, Agita (2005), 'Family policy in Estonia and Latvia', Fafo paper 2005:26, Oslo.

Kerkstra, Ada (1996), 'Netherlands', in Jack B.F. Hutten and Ada Kerkstra (eds), *Home Care in Europe: Country-Specific Guide to its Organization and Financing*, Aldershot: Ashgate, pp. 219–244.

Kerkstra, Ada and Jack B.F. Hutten (1996), 'A cross-national comparison on home care in Europe: summary and findings', in Jack B.F. Hutten and Ada Kerkstra (eds), *Home Care in Europe: Country-Specific Guide to its Organization and Financing*, Aldershot: Ashgate, pp. 1–40.

Kinsella, Kevin and David R. Phillips (2005), 'Global aging: the challenge of success', *Population Bulletin*, **60** (1), 1–42, www.prb.org/pdf05/60.1GlobalAging.pdf, 8 July 2006.

Kitchener, Martin, Terence Ng, Nancy Miller and Charlene Harrington (2005),

'Medicaid home and community-based services: national program trends', *Health Affairs*, **24** (1), 206–12.

Kivisaar, Sirli and Annely Soots (2006), 'The Development of Formal and Informal Care in Estonia', Unpublished report.

Kjær, Anne Mette (2004), *Governance*, Cambridge: Polity.

Klie, Thomas (2004), 'Das personengebundene Budget in den Niederlanden. Ein "wake up call" für die Pflegedienste?' in Thomas Klie and Alexander Spermann (eds), *Persönliche Budgets – Aufbruch oder Irrweg?* Hanover: Vincentz Network, pp. 87–95.

Klie, Thomas and Baldo Blinkert (2002), 'Pflegekulturelle Orientierungen', in Clemens Tesch-Römer (ed.), *Gerontologie und Sozialpolitik*, Stuttgart: Kohlhammer, pp. 197–217.

Knijn, Trudie (1998), 'Social care in the Netherlands', in Jane Lewis (ed.), *Gender, Social Care and Welfare State Restructuring in Europe*, Aldershot: Ashgate, pp. 85–100.

Knijn, Trudie (2000), 'Marketization and the struggling logics of (home) care in the Netherlands', in Madonna Harrington Meyer (ed.), *Care Work: Gender, Labor and the Welfare State*, London and New York: Routledge, pp. 232–48.

Knijn, Trudie (2001), 'Care work: innovations in the Netherlands', in Mary Daly (ed.), *Care Work: The Quest of Security*, Geneva: International Labour Office, pp. 159–74.

Knijn, Trudie (2006), 'Social policy and social interventions: the role of professionals under new governance', Paper presented at the Centre for Comparative Welfare Studies, University of Aalborg, 15 March.

Knijn, Trudie and Monique Kremer (1997), 'Gender and the caring dimension of welfare states: towards inclusive citizenship', *Social Politics*, Fall, 328–61.

Knijn, Trudie and Stijn Verhagen (2003), 'Contested professionalism and the quality of home care', Paper presented at the 6th Conference of the European Sociological Association, Murcia, 22–26 September.

Kooiman, Jan (2000), 'Societal governance: levels, models and orders of social–political interaction', in J. Pierre (ed.), *Debating Governance: Authority, Steering and Democracy*, Oxford: Oxford University Press, pp. 138–64.

Kremer, Monique (2005), 'Consumers in charge of care: the Dutch personal care budget (PGB) and its impact on the market, professionals and the family', unpublished manuscript, The Hague: Netherlands Scientific Council for Government Policy.

Kremer, Monique and Evelien Tonkens (2006), 'Authority, trust, knowledge and the public good in disarray', in Jan Willem Duyvendak, Trudie Knijn and Monique Kremer (eds), *Policy, People, and the New Professional:*

De-Professionalisation and Re-Professionalisation in Care and Welfare, Amsterdam: Amsterdam University Press, pp. 122–34.

Kümpers, Susannne Nicola Sophie (2005), 'Steering integrated care in England and the Netherlands: the case of dementia care. A neo-institutionalist comparative study', PhD Thesis, Department of Health Organisation, Policy and Economics, University of Maastricht, Maastricht.

Lamura, Giovanni, Maria Gabriella Melchiorre, Sabrina Quattrini, Massimo Mengani and Alberto Alberini (2001), 'Background report on Italy', in I. Philp (ed.), *Family Care of Older People in Europe*, Amsterdam: IOS Press, pp. 97–133.

Lamura G., M. Lucchetti and M. Socci (2004), 'Personale straniero e assistenza all'anziano non autosufficiente: due ricerche in Emilia e Marche', in G.A. Micheli (ed.), *I continuanti: interventi a mosaico in una società che invecchia*, Milan: Franco Angeli, pp. 107–26.

Lamura, Giovanni and Francesca Polverini (2005), 'Integrating a multinational workforce in long-term care settings – challenges and opportunities for delivering quality services: lessons from the Italian case', Paper presented at the AARP (American Association of Retired Persons) International Forum on Long Term Care, Washington, DC, 20 October.

Lamura, Giovanni, Francesca Polverini and Maria G. Melchiorre (2006), 'Migrant care workers in long-term care: lessons from the Italian case', Paper presented at the Academy of Health Annual Research Meeting, Seattle, 25–27 June, www.academyhealth.org/2006/607/lamurag.ppt, 10 July 2006.

Land, Hilary and Jane Lewis (1998), 'Gender, care and the changing role of the state in the UK', in Jane Lewis (ed.), *Gender, Social Care and Welfare State Restructuring in Europe*, Aldershot: Ashgate, pp. 51–84.

Landelijke Vereniging van Indicatie Organen (2003), *Werkdocument Gebruikelijk Zorg*, The Hague.

Landenberger, Margarete (1994), 'Pflegeversicherung als Vorbote eines anderen Sozialstaates', *Zeitschrift für Sozialreform*, **40** (3), 314–42.

Landstingsförbundet (2002), *Samarbetet Kring Mediciniskt Färdigbehandlade/Utskrivningsklara Patienter*, Utredningsrapport fran Svenska Kommunförbundet och Landstingsförbundet, Stockholm: Landstingsförbundet.

Leira, Arnlaug and Chiara Saraceno (2003), 'Care: actors, relationships and contexts', in Barbara Hobson, Jane Lewis and Birte Siim (eds), *Contested Concepts in Gender and Social Politics*, Cheltenham, UK and Northampton, MA, USA: Edward Elgar, 55–83.

Lewis, Jane (2001), 'Older people and the health–social care boundary in the UK: half a century of hidden policy conflict', *Social Policy and*

Administration, **35** (4), 343–59.

Lijphart, Arend (1999), *Patterns of Democracy*, New Haven, CT: Yale University Press.

Lovenduski, Joni and Vicky Randall (1993), *Contemporary Feminist Politics: Women and Power in Britain*, Oxford: Oxford University Press.

Low, J.A., W.C. Ng, K.B. Yap and K.M. Chan (2000), 'End-of-life issues: preferences and choices of a group of elderly Chinese subjects', *Annals of the Academy of Medicine*, **29** (1), 50–56.

Lukes, Steven (2005), *Power: A Radical View*, 2nd edn, Basingstoke: Palgrave.

Lundsgaard, Jens (2004a), 'Consumer direction and choice in long-term care for older persons, including payments for informal care. Is it good for care outcomes, employment and fiscal sustainability?', Paper presented at the Symposium: Consumerism of Care for the Elderly, Danish National Institute of Social Research (SFI), Copenhagen, 30 August.

Lundsgaard, Jens (2004b), 'Consumer direction and choice in long-term care for older persons, including payments for informal care: how can it help improve care outcomes, employment and fiscal sustainability?', Health Working Papers 20, Paris: OECD.

Maarse, J.A.M. (1997), 'Netherlands', in Marshall W. Raffel (ed.), *Health Care and Reform in Industrialized Countries*, University Park, PA: Pennsylvania State University Press, pp. 135–62.

Maher, Joanne and Hazel Green (2002), *Carers 2000*, Newcastle-upon-Tyne: National Statistics.

Malin, Nigel (2000), 'Professionalism and boundaries of the formal sector. The example of social and community care', in Nigel Malin (ed.), *Professionalism, Boundaries and the Workplace*, London and New York: Routledge, pp. 7–24.

Matsuda, Shinya (2002), 'The health and social system for the aged in Japan', *Aging Clinical and Experimental Research*, **14** (4), 265–70.

Means, Robin, Sally Richards and Robin Smith (2003), *Community Care: Policy and Practice*, 3rd edn, Basingstoke: Palgrave.

Merlis, Mark (2000), 'Caring for the frail elderly: an international review', *Health Affairs*, **19** (3), 141–9.

Meyer, Jörg Alexander (1996), *Der Weg zur Pflegeversicherung. Positionen, Akteure, Politikprozesse*, Frankfurt am Main: Mabuse Verlag.

Meyer, Martha (2004), 'National Background Report for Germany', EU-Project EUROFAMCARE, Hamburg, www.uke.uni-hamburg.de/EUROFAMCARE, 5 February 2007.

Miltenburg, Theo (2004), 'The impact of personal budgets in the Netherlands', in Thomas Klie and Alexander Spermann (eds), *Persönliche Budgets – Aufbruch oder Irrweg?*, Hanover: Vincentz Network, pp. 81–6.

Ministero dell'Economia e delle Finanze (2006), 'Documento di Programmazione Economica e Finanziaria per gli anni 2007–2011', Rome, www.governo.it/GovernoInforma/documenti_ministeri/dpef2007_2011.pdf, 11 July 2006.

Ministero del Lavoro e delle Politiche Sociali (2005), 'Rapporto di Monitoraggio sulle Politiche Sociali', Rome, www.welfare.gov.it/NR/rdonlyres/eq5sqepebjlruuwyk2xcjlofikiboz3z5vwhhlg2umsay7lct44dpszqvnk2opunrep2cxji3hcs7fv3rlo45qq7h2b/Rapportodimonitoraggiopoliticheso cialius.pdf, 5 February 2007.

Ministero della Salute (2004), 'Rapporto annuale sull'attività di ricovero ospedaliero', Dati SDO 2003, Rome, www.ministerosalute.it/programmazione/sdo/sezDocumenti.jsp?id=102&label=osp, 10 July 2006.

Ministry of Health and Social Affairs (2006), *Nationell utvecklingsplan for vård och omsorg*, Stockholm.

Moran, Michael (1999), *Governing the Health Care State: A Comparative Study of the United Kingdom, the United States and Germany*, Manchester: Manchester University Press.

Moss, Peter and Claire Cameron (2002), *Care Work and the Care Workforce: Report on Stage One and State of the Art Review* (Work Package 6 of 'Care work in Europe. Current understanding and future directions'), London: Institute for Education, University of London.

Naegele, Gerhard (1999), 'The politics of old age in Germany', in Allan Walker and Gerhard Naegele (eds), *The Politics of Old Age in Europe*, Buckingham and Philadelphia, PA: Open University Press, pp. 93–109.

Nahrath, Stéphane (1999), 'The power of ideas in policy research: a critical assessment', in Dietmar Braun and Andreas Busch (eds), *Public Policy and Political Ideas*, Cheltenham, UK and Northampton, MA, USA: Edward Elgar, pp. 41–58.

National Board of Health and Welfare (2000), *Social Services in Sweden in 1999. Needs–Interventions–Development*, Stockholm: National Board of Health and Welfare.

New Zealand Federation of Voluntary Welfare Organisations (2005), '18,000 signature petition for homecare workers', *New Dialogue*, 13 (December), pp. 5–6.

New Zealand Ministry of Health (2000), *The New Zealand Health Strategy*, Wellington: Ministry of Health.

New Zealand Ministry of Health (2002a), *Health of Older People in New Zealand: A Statistical Reference*, Wellington: Ministry of Health.

New Zealand Ministry of Health (2002b), *Health of Older People Strategy: Health Sector Action to 2010 to Support Positive Ageing*, Wellington: Ministry of Health.

New Zealand Ministry of Health (2003), *Achieving Health for All*

People: A Framework for Public Health Action, Wellington: Ministry of Health.

New Zealand Ministry of Health (2006), *Health of Older People Information Strategic Plan: Directions to 2010 and Beyond*, Wellington: Ministry of Health.

New Zealand Ministry for Senior Citizens (2001), *The New Zealand Positive Ageing Strategy*, Wellington: Ministry of Social Policy.

New Zealand Ministry of Social Policy (2001), *The New Zealand Positive Ageing Strategy Action Plan*, Wellington: Ministry of Social Policy.

Newman, Janet (2001), *Modernising Governance*, London: Sage.

Noguchi, Haruko and Satoshi Shimizutani (2005), 'Supplier-induced demand in Japan's at-home care industry', ESRI Discussion Paper Series No. 148, 1–131.

OECD (1966), *Caring for Frail Elderly People. Policies in Evolution*, Social Policy Studies 19, Paris: OECD.

OECD (1988), *OECD Ageing Populations: Social Policy Implications*, Paris: OECD.

OECD (2001), *OECD Health Data 2001. A Comparative Analysis of 30 Countries*, Paris: OECD.

OECD (2004), *OECD Health Data 2004. A Comparative Analysis of 30 Countries*, Paris: OECD.

OECD (2005a), 'OECD in figures', Statistics on the member countries, 2005 edition, Paris: OECD, www.213.253.134.29/oecd/pdfs/browseit/0105061E.PDF, 7 July 2006.

OECD (2005b), *The OECD Health Project: Long-term Care for Older People*, Paris: OECD.

OECD (2006), *Health Data 2006: Statistics and Indicators for 30 Countries*, Paris: OECD.

Österle, August (2001), *Equity Choices and Long-term Care Policies in Europe: Allocating Resources and Burdens in Austria, Italy, the Netherlands and the United Kingdom*, Aldershot: Ashgate.

Ostner, Ilona (1998), 'The politics of care policies in Germany', in Jane Lewis (ed.), *Gender, Social Care and Welfare State Restructuring in Europe*, Aldershot: Ashgate, pp. 111–37.

Øvretveit, J. (1998), *Comparative and Cross-cultural Health Research*, Abingdon, UK: Radcliffe Medical Press.

Pacolet, Jozef, Rita Bouton, Hilde Lanoye and Katia Versieck (2000), *Social Protection for Dependency in Old Age: A Study of Fifteen EU Member States and Norway*, Aldershot: Ashgate.

Palme, Joakim, Åke Bergmark, Olof Bäckmann, Felipe Estrada, Johann Fritzell, Olle Lundberg, Ola Sjöberg, Lena Sommestad and Marta Szebehely (2002), *Welfare in Sweden. The Balance Sheet for the 1990s*,

Ds 2002.32, Stockholm: Ministry of Health and Social Affairs.

Parsons, Wayne (1995), *Public Policy: An Introduction to the Theory and Practice of Policy Analysis*, Cheltenham, UK and Northampton, MA, USA: Edward Elgar.

Pavolini, Emmanuele (2004), *Regioni e politiche sociali per gli anziani. Le sfide della non autosufficienza*, Rome: Carocci Editore.

Pavolini, Emmanuele and Constanzo Ranci (2006), 'Public welfare systems and changes in the demand for welfare: reforms to address chronic needs and the elderly in need of care', Paper presented at the Conference 'European Comparative Research on Ageing – Challenges and Opportunities', Vechta, Germany, 22–24 June.

Per Saldo, www.pgb.nl/showpage.php?pa=3&menu=0,0, 5 February 2007.

Peters, B. Guy (1992), 'The policy process: an institutionalist perspective', *Canadian Public Administration*, **35** (2), 160–80.

Peters, B. Guy (1999), *Institutional Theory in Political Science: The 'New Institutionalism'*, London: Continuum.

Pfau-Effinger, Birgit (2004), *Development of Culture, Welfare State and Women's Employment in Europe*, Aldershot: Ashgate.

Pfau-Effinger, Birgit (2005), 'Development paths of care arrangements in the framework of family values and welfare values', in Birgit Pfau-Effinger and Birgit Geissler (eds), *Care and Social Integration in European Societies*, Bristol: The Policy Press, pp. 21–45.

Pickard, Linda (2001), 'Carer break or carer blind? Policies for informal carers in the UK', *Social Policy and Administration*, **35** (4), 441–58.

Pijl, Marja (2003), *Developments in the Support of Carers: In Finland, England and the Netherlands 1998–2000*, Stockholm: Socialstyrelsen.

Pollitt, C. (2002), 'Clarifying convergence: striking similarities and durable differences in public management reform', *Public Management Review*, **4** (1), 471–92.

Polverini, F. and G. Lamura (2004), 'Labour supply in care services', National Report on Italy, Robert Huggins Associates (RHA), Cardiff (on behalf of the European Foundation for the Improvement of Living and Working Conditions, Dublin), www.assets.aarp.org/www.aarp.org_/articles/GAP/LabourSupplyinCareServices_ItalianReport.pdf, 8 July 2006.

Polverini, Francesca, Andreas Principi, Cristian Balducci, Maria Gaabriella Melchiorre, Sabrina Quattrini, Marie Victoria Gianelli and Giovanni Lamura (2004), *Eurofamcare. National Background Report for Italy*, Ancona: Department of Gerontological Research, Instituto Nazionale di Riposo e Cura Anziani, 'V.E.II'.

Principi, Andrea (2005), 'I trasferimenti monetari nazionali', in Giovanni Lamura, Cristiano Gori, Carlo Hanau, Francesca Polverini, Andrea Principi and Cecilia Tomassini (eds), *L'informazione statistica sull'assistenza agli anziani in Italia. Rapporto di ricerca*, Rome: Presidenza del Consiglio dei Ministri, Commissione di Garanzia per l'Informazione Statistica, pp. 175–95.

Quattrini, Sabrina (2006), 'Main characteristics of the Italian family carers' and older people's sample', in Sabrina Quattrini, Maria Gabriella Melchiorre, Cristian Balducci, Liana Spazzafumo and Giovanni Lamura (eds), *National Survey Report (NASURE): Report on the Main Findings of the EUROFAMCARE Study Survey Carried out in Italy*, Ancona: INRCA, pp. 67–81.

Randall, Vicky (1998), 'Gender and power: women engage the state', in Vicky Randall and Georgina Waylen (eds), *Gender, Politics and the State*, London: Routledge, pp. 185–205.

Randall, Vicky (2000), *The Politics of Childcare in Britain*, Oxford: Oxford University Press.

Rauch, Dietmar (2005), 'Institutional fragmentation and social service variations: a Scandinavian comparison', Doctoral thesis, University of Umeå, Umeå, Sweden.

Robert Wood Johnson Foundation (2001), *A Portrait of Informal Caregivers in America, 2001*, Portland, OR: Foundation for Accountability.

Rosenbrock, Rolf and Thomas Gerlinger (2004), *Gesundheitspolitik. Eine systematische Einführung*, Bern: Hans Huber.

Sabbadini, Linda Laura (2003), 'Donne che curano, donne che vengono curate', in Presidenza del Consiglio dei Ministri, Commissione Nazionale per la Parità e le Pari Opportunità, Curare ed essere curati: una opportunità, un diritto. Atti del Convegno, Milano, 17 January: Istituto Poligrafico e Zecca dello Stato, Rome, pp. 73–92.

Sachverständigenrat für die Konzertierte Aktion im Gesundheitswesen (2001/2002), *Bedarfsgerechtigkeit und Wirtschaftlichkeit*, Vol. 1: *Zielbildung, Prävention, Nutzerorientierung und Partizipation*, Gutachten, www.svr-gesundheit.de/Startseite/Startseite.htm, 5 February 2007.

Saks, Kai, Kristina Oja and Sirli Soots (2003), 'Documentation of Services for the Aged at Risk of Marginalization in Estonia', Report EU-Project CARMA, www.cooss.marche.it/CARMA/, 5 February 2007.

Saltman, Richard B. (1997), 'The context of health reform in the United Kingdom, Sweden, Germany, and the United States', *Health Policy*, **41** (Supplement), S9–S26.

Sand, Ann-Britt M. (2005), 'Informell äldreomsorg samt stöd till informella vårdare – en nordisk forskningsöversikt', in M. Szebehely (ed.), *Äldreomsorgsforskning i Norden, TemaNord 2005:508*, Köpenhamn: Nordiska Ministerrådet, pp. 197–241.

Schmidt, Roland (2002), 'Die neue Pflegelandschaft: Erste Konturen und Steuerungsprobleme', in Clemens Tesch-Römer (ed.), *Gerontologie und*

Sozialpolitik, Stuttgart: Kohlhammer, pp. 137–62.

Schneekloth, Ulrich and Ingo Leven (2003), *Hilfe- und Pflegebedürftige in Privathaushalten in Deutschland 2002*, Munich: Schnellbericht Infratest Sozialforschung.

Schneider, Stu (2003), 'Victories for home health care workers', *Dollars and Sense* (September/October), 25–7.

Schulte, Bernd (1999), 'The legal structures of representation', in Alan Walker and Gerhard Naegele (eds), *The Politics of Old Age*, Buckingham: Open University Press, pp. 25–41.

Schunk, Michaela (1998), 'The social insurance model of care for older people in Germany', in Caroline Glendinning (ed.), *Rights and Realities: Comparing New Developments in Long-Term Care for Older People*, Bristol: Policy Press, pp. 29–46.

Simoni, Simonetta and Rossana Trifiletti (2005), 'Caregiving in transition in Southern Europe: neither complete altruists nor free-riders', in Teppo Kröger and Jorma Sipilä (eds), *Overstretched: European Families up against the Demands of Work and Care*, Oxford: Blackwell, pp. 118–44.

Sipilä, Jorma and Anneli Anttonen (1999), 'Restoring the welfare mix-approach – the ways of producing care', Presentation at the 4th European Conference on Sociology, Amsterdam, 18–21 August.

Skocpol, Theda (1985), 'Bringing the state back in: current research', in Peter B. Evans, Dietrich Rueschemeyer and Theda Skocpol (eds), *Bringing the State Back In*, Cambridge: Cambridge University Press, pp. 3–38.

Sloane, Todd (2005), 'The long-term problem', *Modern Healthcare*, **35** (30), 18.

Socci, Marco, Maria Gabriella Melchiorre, Sabrina Quattrini and Giovanni Lamura (2003), 'Elderly care provided by foreign immigrants: lessons from the Italian case', *Generations Review*, **13** (4), 9–13.

SOS (1999), *Ny lagstiftning om hälso- och sjukvårdspersonalens yrkesbehörigket*, Stockholm: Socialstyrelsen.

SOS (2002), 'Nationell handlingsplan för äldrepolitiken. Slutrapport 2002' (National plan for old age policies. Final report 2002), Stockholm: Socialstyrelsen.

SOS (2003), *Kompetensförsörjning inom vård och omsorg om äldre och funktionshindrade. Del II Faktagrund och beräkningar*, Stockholm: Socialstyrelsen.

SOS (2004), *Etikfrågor i socialtjänsten*, Stockholm: Socialstyrelsen.

SOS (2005a), *Äldre – vård och omsorg år 2004* (Statistik Socialtjänst 2005:2), Stockholm: Socialstyrelsen.

SOS (2005b), *Nya bestämmelser om kvalitet, documentation och anmälningsplikt i lagen* (1993: 397) om stöd och service till vissa funktionshindrade (LSS), m.m. Meddelandeblad Maj 2005, Stockholm:

Socialstyrelsen.
SOSFS (1997a), *Socialstyrelsens allmänna råd. Medicinskt ansvårig sjuksköterska i kommunernas hälso- och sjukvård* (Socialstyrelsens författningssamling, 1997:10), Stockholm: Socialstyrelsen.
SOSFS (1997b), *Socialstyrelsens föreskrifter och allmänna råd: Delegering av arbetsuppgifter inom hälso- och sjukvård och tandvård* (SOSFS, 1997:14), Stockholm: Socialstyrelsen.
SOSFS (1998), *Socialstyrelsens allmänna råd om kvalitetssysem inom omsorgerna om äldre och funktionshindrade* (SOSFS, 1998: 8S), Stockholm: Socialstyrelsen.
SOU (2000), *Samverkansutredning* (SOU, 2000:14), Stockholm: Socialdepartement.
Spence, Ralph (1996), 'Italy', in Ann Wall (ed.), *Health Care Systems in Liberal Democracies*, London: Routledge, pp. 49–76.
Stark, Agneta and Asa Regner (2002), *In Whose Hands? Work, Gender, Ageing and Care in Three EU Countries*, Tema G Report, Linköpings University, Linköping, Sweden.
Statistics New Zealand (2003), *Caregiving, Paid and Unpaid Work*, Wellington: Ministry of Health.
Stone, Robyn I. (2000), *Long-Term Care for the Elderly with Disabilities: Current Policy, Emerging Trends and Implications for the 21st Century*, New York: Milbank Memorial Fund.
Streeck, Wolfgang and Philippe C. Schmitter (1985), 'Community, market, state – and associations? The prospective contribution of interest governance to social order', in Wolfgang Streeck and Philippe C. Schmitter (eds), *Private Interest Government: Beyond Market and State*, Beverly Hills, CA and London: Sage, pp. 1–29.
Szebehely, Marta (1995), *Vardagens organisering*, Lund: Arkiv.
Szebehely, Marta (1996), *Hemhjälp under skiftante villkor – om gamla och hjälpgivare i den svenska hemtjänsten*, Särtryckserien, Stockholm: Socialhögskolan.
Szebehely, Marta (1999a), 'Omsorgsarbete olika former', *Sociologiska Forskning*, **1**, 7–32.
Szebehely, Marta (1999b), 'Concepts and trends in home care for frail elderly people in France and Sweden', in *Comparing Social Welfare Systems in Nordic Europe and France: Copenhagen Conference*, Vol. 4, Paris: Ministère de l'Emploi et de la Solidarité, DREES, MiRe.
Szebehely, Marta (1999c), 'Omsorgsarbetets olika former: Nya klasskillnader och gamla könsmönster i äldreomsorgen', *Sociologisk Forskning*, **36** (1), 7–32.
Szebehely, Marta (2000), 'Äldreomsorg i förändring – knappare resurser och nya organisationsformer', in SOU (2000:38), *Välfärd, vård och och omsorg*,

Antologi/Kommitten Välfärdsbokslut, Stockholm: Social Department, pp. 171–223.

Szebehely, Marta (2005), 'Anhörigas betalda och obetalda äldreomsorgsinsatser', in SOU (2005:66), *Forskingsrapporter till Jämställdhetspolitiska utredningen*, Stockholm: Social Department, pp. 133–203.

Tester, Susan (1996), *Community Care for Older People: A Comparative Perspective*, Basingstoke: Macmillan.

Theobald, Hildegard (2003), 'Care for the elderly: welfare system, professionalisation and the question of inequality', in Birgit Blättel-Mink and Ellen Kuhlmann (eds), Special Issue: Health professions, gender and society. Shifting relations in times of institutional and social change, *International Journal of Sociology and Social Policy*, **23** (4/5), 159–85.

Theobald, Hildegard (2004), 'Care services for the elderly in Germany. Infrastructure, access and utilisation from the perspective of different user groups' (SP I 2004-302), Discussion paper, Working Group on Public Health Policy, Social Science Research Centre (WZB), Berlin.

Theobald, Hildegard (2005), 'Labour market participation of women and social exclusion: contradictory proceses of care employment in Sweden and Germany', in Birgit Pfau-Effinger and Birgit Geissler (eds), *Care and Social Integration in European Societies*, Bristol: Policy Press, pp. 195–213.

Theobald, Hildegard (forthcoming), 'Care arrangements and social integration: the concept of social exclusion and empirical findings in five European countries', Working Paper Series of the Centre for Comparative Welfare Studies, University of Aalborg, Aalborg, Denmark.

Thomas, Carol (1993), 'Deconstructing concepts of care', *Sociology*, **27** (4), 649–69.

Thornley, Carole (2003), 'What future for health care assistants: high road or low road?', in Celia Davies and John Wynn Owen (eds), *The Future Health Workforce*, Basingstoke: Palgrave, pp. 143–60.

Timmermans, Arco (2001), 'Arenas as institutional sites for policymaking: patterns and effects in comparative perspective', *Journal of Comparative Policy Analysis*, **3**, 311–37.

Tinti, Valeria (2004), *Sistema RUG: Risultati Della Prima Rilevazione*, Ancona: Agenzia Regionale Sanitaria Marche.

Tjadens, Frits and Mia Duijnstee (2000), 'The Netherlands', in Frits Tjadens and Marja Pijl (eds), *The Support of Family Carers and Their Organisations in Seven Western-European Countries: State of Affairs in 1998*, Utrecht: Netherlands Institute for Care and Welfare, pp. 71–100.

Tomassini, Cecilia, Karen Glaser, Douglas Wolf, M.I. Broese van Groenou and Emily Grundy (2004), 'Living arrangements among older people: an overview of trends in Europe and the USA', *Population Trends*, **115**, 24–34.

Trifiletti, Rossana (1998), 'Restructuring social care in Italy', in Jane Lewis (ed.), *Gender, Social Care and Welfare State Restructuring in Europe*, Aldershot: Ashgate, pp. 175–206.

Trifiletti, Rossana, Alessandro Pratesi and Simonetta Simoni (2001), 'Care arrangements in dual-career families, National Report: Italy', SOCCARE Project Report 3.3. – WP3, Florence, www.uta.fi/laitokset/sospol/soccare/report3.3.PDF, 5 February 2007.

Trydegard, Gun-Britt (2000), 'Traditions, change and variation: past and present trends in public old-age care', Dissertation, Department of Social Work, University of Stockholm, Stockholm.

Trydegard, Gun-Britt (2003), 'Swedish elderly care in transition: unchanged national policy but substantial changes in practice', Paper presented at the 2003 ESPAnet Conference, Copenhagen, 13–15 November.

Trydegård, G.-B. and M. Thorslund (2001), 'Inequality in the Welfare State? Local variation in care of the elderly – the case of Sweden', *International Journal of Social Welfare*, **10** (3), 174–84.

Twigg, Julia (1989), 'Models of carers: how do social care agencies conceptualise their relationship with informal carers?', *Journal of Social Policy*, **18** (1), 53–66.

Twigg, Julia (1996), 'Issues in informal care', *Caring for Frail Elderly People: Policies in Evolution*, Social Policy Studies 19, OECD, Paris.

Uitvoeringsverslag PGB Nieuwe Stijl (2005), 'Report on personal budgets in the Netherlands', www.cvz.nl/resources/rpt0510_pgb_ns_tcm28-17884.pdf, 5 February 2007.

Ungerson, Clare (ed.) (1990), *Gender and Caring: Work and Welfare in Britain and Scandinavia*, Hemel Hempstead: Harvester Wheatsheaf.

Ungerson, Clare (2003), 'Commodified care work in European labour markets', *European Societies*, **5** (4), 377–96.

Ungerson, Clare (2004), 'Gender, labour markets and care work in five European funding regimes', in Birgit Pfau-Effinger and Birgit Geissler (eds), *Care and Social Integration in European Societies*, Bristol: Policy Press, pp. 49–71.

United Nations, Population Division (1999), 'The world at 6 billions', www.un.org/esa/population/publications/sixbillion/sixbillion.htm, 6 July 2006.

US Department of Health and Human Services (2000), *Informal Caregivers of Disabled Elders with Long-Term Care Insurance*, Washington, DC: Government Printing Office.

US Department of Health and Human Services (2001), *Who Will Care for Us? Addressing the Long-Term Care Workforce Crisis*, Washington, DC:

Government Printing Office.

US Department of Health and Human Services (2003), *Promising Practices in the Field of Caregiving*, Washington, DC: Government Printing Office.

US Department of Health and Human Services (2004), *Recent Findings on Frontline Long-Term Care Workers*, Washington, DC: Government Printing Office.

Vabo, Mia (2004), 'Consumer power: increasing choice for recipients?', Paper presented at the symposium on Consumerism of Care for the Elderly, Danish National Institute of Social Research (SFI), Copenhagen, 20 August 2004.

Vabo, Mia (2005), 'New Public Management i nordisk eldreomsorg – hva forskes det på?', in Marta Szebehely (ed.), *Äldreomsorgsforskning i Norden. En kunskapsöversikt*, Tema Nord 2005:508, Köpenhamn: Nordiska ministerrådet, pp. 73–111.

Verhagen, Stijn (2005), *Zorglogica's uit balans. Het onbehagen in de thuiszorg nader verklaard*, Utrecht: de Graaf.

Vidler, Elizabeth and John Clarke (2005), 'Creating citizen-consumers: New Labour and the remaking of public services', *Public Policy and Administration*, **20** (2), 19–37.

Visser-Jansen, G. and C.P.M. Knipscheer (2004), *Eurofamcare: National Background Report for the Netherlands*, Amsterdam: Free University.

Waerness, Kari (1984), 'The rationality of caring', *Economic and Industrial Democracy*, **5**, 185–211.

Walker, Allan (1999), 'Political participation and representation of older people', in Alan Walker and Gerhard Naegele (eds), *The Politics of Old Age*, Buckingham: Open University Press, pp. 7–24.

Wasem, Jürgen (1997), 'A study of decentralizing from acute care to home care settings in Germany', *Health Policy*, **41** (Supplement), S109–29.

Waylen, Georgina (1998), 'Gender, feminism and the state: an overview', in Vicky Randall and Georgina Waylen (eds), *Gender, Politics and the State*, London: Routledge, pp. 1–17.

Welti, Felix (1999a), 'Vorbehaltene Aufgabenbereiche für Pflegeberufe', Part 1, *Pflege- und Krankenhausrecht*, **2**, Vol. 2/99, 29–33.

Welti, Felix (1999b), 'Vorbehaltene Aufgabenbereiche für Pflegeberufe', Part 3, *Pflege- und Krankenhausrecht*, **2**, Vol. 4/99, 85–90.

Wenger, Eldon L. (2001), 'Restructuring care for the elderly in Germany', *Current Sociology*, **49** (3), 175–88.

Wenger, Jonathan (2004), 'At-home care for elderly gaining favor', *Omaha World-Herald,* 6 December, p. A3.

Wilensky, Gail R. (2005), 'The challenges of Medicaid', *Healthcare Financial Management*, **59** (6), 34–5.

Witz, Anne (1990), 'Patriarchy and professions: the gendered politics of occupational closure', *Sociology*, **24** (4), 675–90.

Wrede, Sirpa, Cecilia Benoit and Jane Sandall (2001), 'The state and birth/the state of birth: maternal health policy in three countries', in Raymond De Vries, Cecilia Benoit, Edwin R. van Tejlingen and Sirpa Wrede (eds), *Birth by Design: Pregnancy, Maternity Care, and Midwifery in North America and Europe*, New York and London: Routledge.

Zeman, Peter (2005), 'Pflege in familiärer Lebenswelt', in Klaus R. Schroeter and Thomas Rosenthal (eds), *Soziologie der Pflege*, Weinheim: Juventa, pp. 247–62.

Index